Praise for *Breaking Canadians*

"These unique voices tell stories from the home, the schools, and the bedsides chronicling a litany of suffering, neglect, and outright public health negligence. *Breaking Canadians* is a rallying call to ensure we fix what is broken in our public health care system."

Cathy Crowe, long-time street nurse, C.M.

"The story of Canada's experience with – and response to – COVID-19 is only now starting to be written. Every one of us has a valid perspective. But the recollections of those prominently on the front lines of medical treatment, outbreak management, patient advocacy, and public engagement are, to my mind, the most useful. *Breaking Canadians* is a collection of perspectives from prominent Canadian patient advocates whose names became well known during the pandemic. The essays are not dry academic expositions, but rather personal evocations embracing a host of accessible emotions – most commonly frustration and disappointment. But sprinkled here and there are seeds of hope, as kernels of policy insight also emerge to answer that all important question: what do we do next?"

Raywat Deonandan, Epidemiologist and Professor, University of Ottawa

"Dr. Nili Kaplan-Myrth has been a fierce, unwavering, and courageous advocate for the well-being of patients and citizens throughout the COVID-19 pandemic. In *Breaking Canadians*, she has assembled dozens of Canadian voices that must be heard to appreciate the ongoing burden of the worst public health event in living memory. From the testimonies of those most affected, to the contributions of advocates and scholars, *Breaking Canadians* documents how very much has gone wrong and illuminates a path forward towards greater public safety, equity, and respectful engagement."

Robert Maunder, Chair in Health and Behaviour, Sinai Health, and Professor of Psychiatry, University of Toronto

"*Breaking Canadians* focuses an unflinching gaze on the COVID-19 pandemic. Perhaps its most devastating revelation is that scientists concluded within the *first two months* that the virus spread by aerosol transmission, *not* by droplets or dirty groceries. Yet our governments serially dropped masking requirements, avoided installing air filters, and withheld crucial data from the public. We should all read this book and reflect."

Jan Wong, Journalist and Author of *Red China Blues* and *Apron Strings*

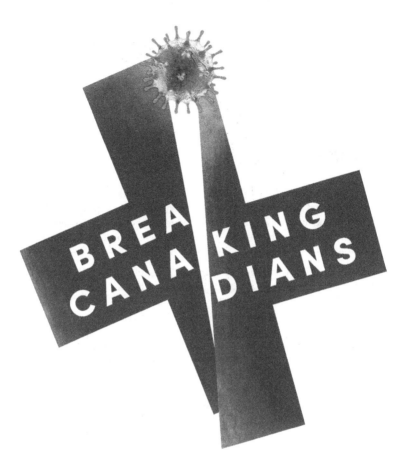

HEALTH CARE, ADVOCACY, AND THE TOLL OF COVID-19

EDITED BY

NILI KAPLAN-MYRTH, MD, PHD

ÆVO UTP

Aevo UTP
An imprint of University of Toronto Press
Toronto Buffalo London
utorontopress.com
© Nili Kaplan-Myrth 2023

ISBN 978-1-4875-4812-4 (paper)   ISBN 978-1-4875-4813-1 (EPUB)
                                        ISBN 978-1-4875-4814-8 (PDF)

Library and Archives Canada Cataloguing in Publication
Title: Breaking Canadians : health care, advocacy, and the toll of
COVID-19 / edited by Nili Kaplan-Myrth, MD, PhD.
Names: Kaplan-Myrth, Nili, editor.
Description: Includes bibliographical references.
Identifiers: Canadiana (print) 20230552137 | Canadiana (ebook) 20230552161 |
ISBN 9781487548124 (paper) | ISBN 9781487548148 (PDF) |
ISBN 9781487548131 (EPUB)
Subjects: LCSH: COVID-19 Pandemic, 2020 – Canada. | LCSH: Medical care –
Canada. | LCSH: Equality – Canada.
Classification: LCC RA644.C67 B74 2024 | DDC 362.1962/414400971 – dc23

Cover design: Sandra Friesen
Cover image: iStock.com/ffikretow

We wish to acknowledge the land on which the University of Toronto Press
operates. This land is the traditional territory of the Wendat, the Anishnaabeg, the
Haudenosaunee, the Métis, and the Mississaugas of the Credit First Nation.

University of Toronto Press acknowledges the financial support of the Government
of Canada, the Canada Council for the Arts, and the Ontario Arts Council, an
agency of the Government of Ontario, for its publishing activities.

Canada Council   Conseil des Arts
for the Arts   du Canada

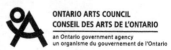

ONTARIO ARTS COUNCIL
CONSEIL DES ARTS DE L'ONTARIO
an Ontario government agency
un organisme du gouvernement de l'Ontario

Funded by the   Financé par le
Government   gouvernement
of Canada   du Canada

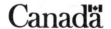

Contents

Foreword   ix
DR. BRIAN GOLDMAN

Introduction: I Can't. I'm Too Broken   1
DR. NILI KAPLAN-MYRTH

PART I: IN THE COMMUNITY   25

1 Casualty   27
   LYNDA HURLEY

2 Pandemic, Alone   29
   LEORA EISEN

3 Present Tense   34
   TANIA J. SPENCER

4 A Community Divided   41
   ANONYMOUS

5 BC – Breaking Cancer   45
   DR. JAIGRIS HODSON

6 Learning to Count   49
   ELEANOR RAMPHAL

7 The Spring   52
   DR. DAVID KEEGAN

PART II: AT THE MARGINS   61

8 Long-Term Care or Long-Term Crime?   63
   DR. VIVIAN STAMATOPOULOS

9 Go Home   85
   KIMIKO SHIBATA

10 Ableism   93
   KENZIE McCURDY

11 Still Here   98
   REVEREND CANON MAGGIE HELWIG

12 The Pandemic Changed Nothing (for Worse
   and Better)   102
   MEAGAN GILLMORE

13 Wild Teens: Youth Mental Health
   and the Pandemic   113
   DR. GAIL BECK

14 The Pandemic Ends ... Then What?   124
   ANNIE LIN

PART III: THE CRUMBLING BASE — 129

15 Resilience Is a Dirty Word — 131
DEBRA LEFEBVRE

16 Men Write the Policies, Women Face the Results — 142
DR. MICHELLE COHEN

17 #InItTogether Is Only a Hashtag for Canadian Caregivers — 160
MAGGIE KERESTECI

18 Invisible — 166
SARAH KAPLAN

19 The Levee Has Broken — 174
KIM ENGLISH

PART IV: NO SIMPLE FIXES — 181

20 "We're All in This Together": COVID-19 and Principles of Environmental Justice — 183
DR. JANE E. McARTHUR

21 This Ain't No Flu — 198
DR. STEVE FLINDALL

22 The Doctor as Advocate — 209
DR. JOE VIPOND

23 Disability Rights and Advocacy — 220
DR. CHRISTOPHER LEIGHTON

24 "Truth"   231
DR. IMOGEN COE

25 I Work in a Hospital. You Are an Internet Troll.
We Are Not the Same   243
DR. GENEVIEVE EASTABROOK

26 How to Be Wrong: Reflections on the (Non)
Evolution of Applied Medical Science during
Epidemics   251
DR. DAVID FISMAN

Postscript: Roll Up Your Sleeves   271
SUE ROBINS

Notes   277

Foreword

DR. BRIAN GOLDMAN

Do you remember where you were when the World Health Organization (WHO) declared COVID-19 a pandemic? Like many Canadians, my memories are fragmented and blurred.

Utah Jazz forward Rudy Gobert tested positive for the virus. Within hours, the National Basketball Association suspended its schedule. At almost the same moment on the other side of the world, actor Tom Hanks and his partner Rita Wilson became the most famous twosome on the planet to be infected.

As host of the CBC Radio program *White Coat, Black Art*, my team of producers and I were ordered to work from home. It would be another two years before I returned to my office to gather some things.

If we stayed in our own protective bubbles, for the most part, we were safe. But the safety we gained came at a terrible cost. Removed from in-person gatherings, we began to spend too much time in our heads and not enough in our hearts. We lost the capacity for empathy. The empathy was replaced by fear.

That was not the case in the ER at Sinai Health System, where I've worked for decades. In the first waves of the pandemic, we drew together in kindness and solidarity.

In my first night shift at the start of the pandemic, my friend and ER colleague, Dr. Paul Koblic, pulled me aside for a private chat. Paul was working the "casino" shift from 9 p.m. to 3 or 4 a.m., depending on how busy the ER would be.

"If any of your patients need intubation, I'll do them for you," he whispered.

Back then, we had a disease with a name, no vaccine, and no evidence-based treatments. We also had a lot of very bad memories of the SARS outbreak in 2003, which preyed upon healthcare workers in close contact with infected patients. Some of our colleagues back then ended up on ventilators, and some of them died.

Fortunately, no one arrived that night who needed intubation. I never forgot Paul's gesture of selfless kindness.

Within weeks, Paul and my other colleagues created new step-by-step protocols for Protected Code Blues (PCBs) that enabled front-line healthcare workers like us to take care of patients with severe COVID-19 pneumonia without endangering ourselves and others. We shot how-to videos and did endless simulated resuscitations.

There was palpable nervous energy in the air as we hunkered down to meet the crisis. Maybe it's that we never stopped going to work. I can recall times when I was happy to be going to work in the ER because it meant I would be around colleagues in a collective struggle against a ghastly but (hopefully) winnable virus.

And we were celebrated by our patients and by society at large. Every night at 7:30 p.m., grateful citizens stood outside on street corners and balconies and banged pots in celebration of front-line healthcare workers.

As we know all too well, that nightly celebration morphed into anger at public health, politicians, and us. The rules put in place to protect our most vulnerable citizens became unbearable to those not affected directly by the virus.

You can argue against the maladaptive and sometimes criminal actions taken by some. What you can't argue or rationalize away are the feelings that led to those actions.

COVID-19 and the social and economic dislocations that it caused have put our society under stress. The mental health implications of the pandemic that include depression, anxiety, substance use, and self-harm are and will be present for years if not decades to come.

Human beings have two diverging and contradictory aspects to our nature. We are hardwired to be empathic to others. We have dual-purpose neurons that light up when we complete an act of kindness and light up when we observe someone else carrying out the same action. Neuroscientists believe these dual-purpose neurons (called mirror neurons) are the seat of empathy. These cells reside in our frontal lobes where we use judgment and reason to guide our actions.

Newborns first experience kindness from their parents. The hormone oxytocin prepares the womb to give birth, the breast to give life-sustaining milk, and the heart of a new mother to adore her children. That is the beginning of the attachment bond between parent and child that is essential to raising offspring to the point at which they can care for themselves and restart the cycle.

Without that attachment, humans would not build neighbourhoods and communities and do good works for perfect strangers. Without it, we would kill ourselves many times over.

But empathy and kindness are only half of our nature. Deep inside our primitive brains lies the seat of something else: a nubbin of brain cells that decides for us if a stranger is a friend or a foe. That part of the brain detects signals from physical characteristics, body posture, skin colour, language, vocabulary, and even tone of voice. Within mere nanoseconds, our brains tell us either to invite the stranger into our homes or lock the door and grab the nearest weapon.

In normal times, we are governed by the higher centres that reside in our frontal lobes. Our frontal lobes override the primitive instinct to designate strangers as enemies.

Our brains have an Achilles' heel, and that is stress. The catecholamines that bathe our minds when we are stuck in traffic or on an airport tarmac waiting hours to deplane take our frontal lobes offline. That leaves our primitive selves in charge.

Our society is in the grip of pandemic stress. Our primitive selves seem to be in charge. We have lost the kindness and empathy that make us human. Laid low by societal anger and by some politicians who take their service for granted, healthcare workers are burning out and quitting in record numbers.

The path to re-establishing empathy as our go-to response to human suffering is by tackling head on the stress that continues to grip us. That is the only way that we will once again see others as friends and not as bitter enemies.

We need to take the stress out of our daily lives. The most effective way to do that across society is to carefully build the social safety net. Almost certainly, that means redistributing wealth through taxation and social programs.

Instead of aiming our pandemic stress at perceived opponents, we need to channel it into effective action. As a wealthy society, we have the means to reduce the stress of disadvantaged members of society by addressing the socio-economic determinants of health. Better housing, better access to green grocers, and adequate sick leave will do much to relieve the stressors that were exacerbated during the pandemic.

This book is necessary now because it recognizes those needs and because it provides a pathway to effective action.

All we need is the will to see it through. Our very existence as a caring society is what's at stake.

BRIAN GOLDMAN, MD, CFPC (EM), is a staff emergency physician at the Schwartz Reisman Emergency Centre at Sinai Health System. He is the host of *White Coat, Black Art* on CBC Radio One, and the host of the CBC podcast *The Dose*. His latest book – *The Power of Teamwork: How We Can All Work Better Together* – was published in 2022.

Introduction

I Can't. I'm Too Broken

DR. NILI KAPLAN-MYRTH

"Our healthcare system is decimated … This government's callous treatment of every healthcare worker has us holding on by the slimmest of threads. It is only because of the dedication and caring of the remaining healthcare workers that we are still functioning at our current level."
– Anonymous public health professional, Ontario, 2022

"We have learned nothing."
– Anonymous epidemiologist, 2022

"Even if Covid-19 is real … you people are just so confused in the head by watching mainstream media pouring their lies into your ears and you listen to every lying word … we're not their slaves."
"Even if Covid-19 is real? Where the hell have you been living for the last 3 years?"
– Twitter exchange between two people, 2022

It is 1 October 2022, as I sit down to write this introduction. The Government of Canada reports more than 17,000 new cases of COVID-19 in the past week, and 196 more deaths.[1] Since the beginning of the pandemic, that brings the total number of recorded COVID-19 cases to 4,233,468 across Canada, and the total number of deaths to 44,992. Given waste-water levels and other indicators (workplace absences, critical understaffing of healthcare and other occupations and industries), it is reasonable to assume that we have grossly underestimated the spread and impact of COVID-19 in our communities over the course of two and a half years. For certain, the raw numbers do nothing to capture the long-term toll that this disease will have on Canadians, or the disproportionate effects of the pandemic on our most vulnerable populations: Black, Indigenous, and racialized people, financially insecure populations, seniors, young children, people with disabilities, and women.

On each occasion that I sit down to work on *Breaking Canadians* – sometimes a lapse of weeks, sometimes months – it feels more difficult to capture our specific moment in time.

At the beginning of the pandemic, I stepped up to speak publicly about the impact of COVID-19 on primary care providers and our patients. I joined conversations with colleagues and community members, through radio, television, print media, and social media.

Early on, it felt like perhaps we were "in this together," at least insofar as we were all focused on survival and unsure of our future. That unity quickly gave way to a competition for resources: people scrambled for toilet paper, then for hand sanitizer and personal protective equipment (PPE).

When the "hunt" began in earnest for vaccines, I organized a roundtable discussion about inequities in the vaccine roll-out with Prime Minister Trudeau and the federal minister of health, Patty Hajdu.

Today, it is worse than a lack of unity or even a competition for resources. Today, it feels like there is a total disconnect between the reality of COVID-19 and the general public's perception of COVID-19. For healthcare professionals, people with long COVID, people who are immunocompromised or have disabilities, people who have lost a loved one to COVID-19, and people who are still doing their damnedest to avoid this disease, there is a sense of betrayal that politicians and policymakers have abandoned all preventative measures and have recklessly opened the floodgates for mass-infection. COVID-19 still profoundly shapes my work and life as a family physician. Every day, we have multiple patients who are (re)infected, some with serious consequences. Non-healthcare professionals, in contrast, are by and large under the illusion that COVID-19 is over. They are not to blame. Lack of transparency in communication from public health leaders and from politicians, the ever-shifting, always confusing policies and procedures around COVID-19, and the media's role in giving a voice to people who spread disinformation have all contributed to the situation we find ourselves in today.

A small number of colleagues with their own political and ideological lenses are pushing a narrative of "freedom," equating public health preventative measures with "restrictions." A growing cadre of hateful people with anti-science, anti-mask, anti-vaxx, and anti-democracy agendas is waiting in the wings to attack whatever my esteemed colleagues (many of them with pieces in *Breaking Canadians*) say, to belittle us, harass us with more threats, and embolden racism, misogyny, antisemitism, homophobia, and transphobia.

It is not an easy time to be an advocate for the health and well-being of the community, to stand up for marginalized and vulnerable populations. Indeed, it is not a good time to be outspoken as a Canadian healthcare professional – or a journalist, or a politician – particularly if one is a woman, Black, Indigenous, racialized, Jewish, 2SLGBTQ+, or a person with disabilities.

Where will we all be when this goes to publication? Where will you be when you read this? How will you receive people's stories of their experiences of the pandemic?

In part, writing *Breaking Canadians* is a challenge because the last few years are such a blur. We've lost our sense of time, and our current timeline feels so surreal. I can't recall each twist and turn, from late 2019 when the first known SARS-CoV-2 infection was identified in Wuhan, China, to 25 January 2020, the first identified case in Canada, to 11 March 2020, when the World Health Organization declared a pandemic. I can only offer snapshots of key themes and pivotal moments between March 2020 and October 2022, from my perspective as a family physician working and living in central Ottawa, Canada's capital city. Travel back with me to the first eight months of the pandemic when, in October 2020, I wrote a brief timeline for the *Ottawa Citizen*, which is adapted here:[2]

In March 2020, I was afraid because my patients were coughing so hard they couldn't speak, were so tired they couldn't get out of bed. We didn't know how to help them. We huddled around our radio and listened to Prime Minister Trudeau urge Canadians to come home from abroad. Friends and family crossed back into Canada just before the border closed. I saw colleagues in healthcare – doctors, nurses, PSWs – dying in Hubei province and Rome and New York City. I panicked because I didn't have a will. I was afraid because there was controversy about whether masks were helpful, and nobody understood what it meant to maintain physical distance or form social bubbles. We didn't know how we'd survive, financially or socially. People were trapped on cruises. Schools closed and didn't reopen for the academic year. We were in free-fall.

In April 2020, COVID-19 dominated my life. As a family doctor in the community, I had no personal protective equipment, and I didn't know how I would be able to continue to care for my patients. In Ontario, many doctors had to wait to be paid from March to July, as the Ministry of Health established new billing codes for virtual care. Across Canada, colleagues struggled to keep our clinics from closing, we pivoted to telemedicine/video. I answered calls to patients 24/7, wrote articles, reached out to media. We were called "heroes," but we already felt demoralized, exhausted. I stared at my computer waiting for advice from our medical organizations. COVID-19 dominated my life as I tried to manage my patients' mental health and physical health and realized I wouldn't see extended family for a long time.

I was afraid of COVID-19 in May 2020, as some of my patients who were sick in March and April got sicker. We still had little capacity for testing, almost no tracing. I was afraid as my patients with disabilities were locked into their assistive living homes, asking me why they had lost their freedom. My patients in hospital and long-term care (LTC) weren't allowed to have their loved ones at their sides. I watched in horror as more than 81 per cent of deaths were in LTC, and staff abandoned those facilities. I was forlorn as I watched women disproportionately leave their jobs to take on childcare. I was worried as children with learning disabilities and special education needs struggled with home schooling. I was afraid as domestic violence put my patients, trapped in their homes, at greater risk. I was sad when we witnessed George Floyd's murder, and we had to put on our masks and hit the streets in protest.

COVID-19 dominated my life in June 2020, as even though millions participated in Black Lives Matter rallies, we knew that racism was rampant in our own backyard in Canada. We acknowledged that there were higher death rates in poorer neighbourhoods, and that Indigenous populations, people of colour, and other marginalized groups were disproportionately affected by this pandemic, but we weren't collecting sufficient race-based and socio-economic data. COVID-19 dominated my life as I watched my patient's father die of neglect in LTC, from bed sores that could have been treated if his essential caregivers had been allowed to care for him.

I was afraid of COVID-19 in July 2020, as only the most privileged segment of our population had access to green spaces. I was afraid as our governments moved from one phase of policy to another, and people started to have a cavalier attitude about their social bubbles. I swore that I wouldn't eat in a restaurant, go out to a pub, or get my hair cut before we knew that we had plans to ensure it would be safe for schools to open in September. I was afraid again for my colleagues as we learned that a doctor in the US committed suicide from the post-traumatic stress of running an emergency room.

In August 2020, educators demanded plans for September, but we all knew that there was no plan to ensure safety in classrooms. COVID-19 dominated my life as groups of drunken young adults cycled past me on mobile bars, and I yelled at them to put on masks. COVID dominated my life as I gradually opened my office for more in-person visits and tried to figure out how to focus again on chronic illnesses and preventative medicine.

In September 2020, I was ashamed of our healthcare system as Joyce Echaquan's death highlighted institutionalized racism. Systemic inequalities were all around us, as privileged parents chose to withdraw from public education, forming private pods. I was worried when COVID-19 testing centres were overwhelmed and dismayed as I watched my patients form long lines, standing for hours with sick children in their arms. People with disabilities couldn't access tests. People started to pay huge sums for private tests. I was afraid when I received a memo from our local public health unit to say that we should have a "low threshold for testing," reminding us that we cannot distinguish clinically between COVID and other respiratory illnesses. I was even more afraid in the following weeks, as our public health guidelines inexplicably changed, and we couldn't separate politics from sound policy. I was afraid and upset when we were notified that there was a case of COVID in my own child's classroom. I was afraid because everyone needs the ability to test, paid sick leave, small classrooms, access to care.

In October 2020, COVID-19 dominated my life as I watched the president of the United States parading around without a mask, contagious, saying that he is not scared. COVID-19 dominated my life because we could not rely on public health transparency. COVID-19 dominated my life as I faced sexism speaking as a female physician on live national television. COVID-19 dominated my life as I told my children and patients that the idea of "social bubbles" had burst. I joined my colleagues in yelling from the rooftop that we need to act before it's too late. Some patients who were sick in March 2020 were still unwell.

COVID-19 dominated our children's lives, as school outbreaks left children bouncing back and forth between virtual platforms and actual classrooms; they couldn't safely participate in extracurricular activities; they were asked not to gather with their friends. The concept of "long COVID" had not yet emerged. We urged politicians and public health officials to think about the cost of morbidity (illness), not just death. COVID-19 dominated my life as I warned that the lack of testing and tracing will falsely make it look as though numbers go down, justifying our government's inaction. COVID-19 dominated my life as cases were surging, the second wave hit, hard, and there was no end in sight.

Fast forward to spring 2021. We watched as people died by the thousands and were loaded into refrigerated trucks in New York City. We watched as field hospitals were set up in Canadian cities. We monitored daily data on COVID-19 infections, hospital, long-term care (LTC), and school outbreaks, death counts, and vaccine uptake. We watched in horror as stories of neglect emerged from LTC facilities across Canada and we raised alarm bells as personal support workers (PSWs) died without masks and migrant workers died in farmers' fields. We shook our heads as the "heroes" who work on the front line begged for more PPE and doctors' clinics in our communities closed because of a lack of provincial support. We were pleased when the people shelving groceries were offered "pandemic pay" and then dismayed when their small bonuses were clawed back. We waited patiently for COVID-19 PCR testing to become widely available, and then became despondent as those same testing centres closed their doors and most reporting and tracing disappeared. We advocated for Rapid Antigen Tests (RATs) to be distributed to every child and educator, then called out our provinces for providing them to private schools before public schools. We begged for masks to be universally mandated, then watched as they were blithely discarded. We stood up for the most vulnerable sectors of our populations, went above and beyond for our patients and communities, and then we – physicians, nurses, health advocates – became the recipients of death threats, the targets of racism and misogyny and hate for stepping onto a public stage.

"You are not broken, the system is broken," I said that spring, when I put out the call for submissions for *Breaking Canadians*. I was speaking to the doctors, nurses, educators, grocers, construction workers, childcare providers, essential caregivers, and others who reached out to me to say, "I can't. I'm too broken."

In late summer 2021, I gathered a group of healthcare professionals and educators outside of city hall in Ottawa and at Queen's Park in Toronto to ask provincial politicians and policymakers to prepare for a safe September. We had all the knowledge and tools to prevent the spread of a disease that we had watched ravage our population. Epidemiologists globally were calling for an acknowledgment that COVID-19 is airborne, and explaining that we needed to upgrade the masks we wore to N95s/respirators, that we needed to improve ventilation and use HEPA filtration systems in indoor spaces, and that COVID-19 vaccines would reduce serious illness, hospitalization, and death. The Province of Ontario's Science Table released an advisory: "Our models, federal models, and models in other jurisdictions predict a substantial 4th wave. Vaccination offers substantial protection against severe health outcomes. We do not expect to see the same proportion of severely ill cases in the vaccinated. Among the unvaccinated, we do expect to see a rapid increase in the number of seriously ill people needing hospital care as workplaces and education re-open in September. The fourth wave will affect all age groups with the potential to exceed ICU capacity."[3]

At that time, Canada was engrossed in a federal election. A man was arrested for throwing stones at Justin Trudeau's campaign. Anti-maskers and anti-vaxxers began staging protests outside of hospitals in Toronto, Montreal, Vancouver, and other cities and rural settings across the country. These "protestors" asserted that they were angry about vaccine mandates, but their slogans and flags, as they harassed healthcare professionals and blocked ambulances and patients from accessing care, were dog-whistles for populist, white supremacist groups. I ended my speech outside of Queen's Park with the words, "There is no place for hate in our streets."

Between February 2021 and November 2021, like many of my racialized and female colleagues, I became a target for death threats because I was speaking in support of public health measures and tools. The "Jabapalooza" community vaccine clinics that I organized first for my own patients and then for essential workers, people with disabilities, educators, and pregnant people in Ottawa responded to a dire need in the community, to ensure that people would not have to "hunt" for vaccines. We gave approximately 20,000 doses of vaccine through dozens of clinics, run in the Ottawa Footy Sevens' soccer field, in the corridors of TD Place, in neighbourhood elementary and secondary schools, and on the street in front of my clinic. We did it all with an incredible team of volunteers. Ottawa Chamberfest played at a clinic, as dark clouds rolled across the sky and people cried tears of relief to get their COVID-19 vaccines. My work was celebrated (I was the "News Maker of the Year" of 2021, according to the *Ottawa Citizen*), but it also made me the focus of worsening harassment on social media and in the community.

In December 2021, Dr. Katharine Smart, the president of the Canadian Medical Association, came to my clinic to bring me a bouquet of flowers during a junior Jabapalooza. She wanted to let me know that on 17 December 2021, Bill

C-3 would be passed in the House of Commons to amend the Criminal Code, which would make it an offence to intimidate or impede a patient from seeking care, or to intimidate or impede a healthcare professional from performing their duties.

Then, on 22 January 2022, a hate-fuelled convoy rolled into the streets of downtown Ottawa with Confederate flags and swastikas and Fuck Trudeau signs draped on their trucks, in the guise of an "anti-vaccine mandate" protest, but with a stated position that their intention was to overthrow our democratically elected government. While horns blared at all hours and Ottawa's downtown population was traumatized by convoy participants, encampments were set up outside of the city, and weapons were seized at a US–Canadian border crossing, the media took photographs of bouncy castles in front of Parliament Hill. The veneer of "fun" was eventually replaced by an acknowledgment that there was nothing humorous about the harassment of Ottawa citizens by racist, anti-science, and anti-democratic disruptors. In an open letter signed by more than 2,000 healthcare professionals across Canada, which was sent to the mayor of Ottawa, the premiers of every province and territory, and the prime minister, we again asserted, "There is no place for hate in our streets."

On 14 February 2022, the Emergencies Act was invoked by the Government of Canada, and the convoy was forced out of downtown Ottawa. A subsequent enquiry into the Ottawa Police's response to the occupation included the revelation that there were sympathetic elements within the police force. Despite all of this, municipal, provincial, and federal politicians who emboldened the occupation of Ottawa, and local businesses that supported the convoy, were unapologetic. Worse still, their rhetoric of "freedom" slipped into mainstream discourse. Then the fourth wave of COVID-19 hit, followed by a fifth wave, and sixth wave, and Canadian media continued to give voice to people who minimized the significance of COVID-19 on children, who dismissed the existence of long COVID, and who pushed for a "new normal."

Fast forward again to spring 2022. COVID-19 variants Alpha, Beta, Gamma, and Delta were overtaken by a highly transmissible new variant, Omicron, as our public health units across Canada declared that we were entering the seventh wave of the COVID-19 pandemic. Meanwhile, politicians across the country and around the world, in a bizarre capitulation to the rhetoric of anti-maskers, anti-vaxxers, and far-right political movements, declared that Omicron was "mild," and it was "time to move on." Sports and entertainment and other industries encouraged Canadians to "return to normal."

In Canada and elsewhere, there was a general chorus of people raising alarms, begging our leaders to acknowledge that the latest variant was no joke, that infants and kids were getting sick in larger numbers, and that health policy was fraught with ableism, ageism, racism, and disregard for the most vulnerable in our populations. Epidemiologists and public health professionals warned us early in the pandemic that provincial medical directives weren't sufficient, that policies weren't keeping up with science, and that our populations were in trouble. Across Canada and around the world, public health measures were thrown out, vaccine mandates were discarded rather than updated, and masks were discarded rather than updated. Political directives were sent to public health units to stop collecting data. Reporting of cases in schools or elsewhere stopped, as though we could look the other way and this problem would disappear. Hospitals across Canada, particularly in rural areas, were so critically understaffed in the summer of 2022 that emergency rooms, community medical clinics, and family medicine offices closed.

Nobody with the power to act cared.

Although most Canadians were willing to roll up their sleeves for the COVID-19 vaccine and most children and adults would have happily continued to mask in public spaces, the messages of a small number of anti-vaxxers and anti-maskers powerfully undermined health policy and politics. There are those of us who have advocated throughout the pandemic that safety should not be a privilege, that all along we should have talked about our tools for preventing COVID-19 as "protections," not "restrictions." Then there are those who talk about masks as though they are an "infringement of freedom," physicians and nurses who spread disinformation about vaccines, those who still want to quibble about whether people are hospitalized "with" or "because of" COVID-19, who feel no moral qualm with making policy decisions and personal decisions that adversely and irreversibly affect others. Public health isolation rules were shortened from ten days to five days, and then discarded altogether, and contagious employees were encouraged to return to workplaces. Although that was a decision based on critical staff shortages, the layperson was misled to believe that there was no longer a "risk" associated with COVID-19. Medical officers of health made no effort to challenge politicians and media who told us that it is time to get "back to normal." Epidemiologists, physicians, nurses, other healthcare workers, caregivers, childcare providers, and educators were gaslit by some politicians when they cried foul.

It took longer than a year for medical institutions and governments to acknowledge that COVID-19 is airborne, and even then there was no concerted effort to reach out to the public with this message, not because of the science but because of the politics; initially, the focus was on droplet spread and it was easier to continue to tell people to wash hands and sterilize surfaces than to speak transparently about the need for better ventilation and higher-level masks and all the infrastructural implications. Similarly, COVID-19 vaccine mandates focused on two doses as "fully vaccinated." Rather than update the requirements to include booster doses, based on evidence of waning immunity, politicians undermined immunization programs by lifting vaccine requirements.

All of which brings us to where we are (as I write this today) in October 2022, almost three years since the beginning of the global COVID-19 pandemic. Some of us aren't ready to shrug off what we see as an ongoing tragedy. Some of us are still grieving the more than 6.5 million lives worldwide lost to COVID-19. Some of us are worried about long-term consequences of more than 600 million people worldwide infected with a virus that may irreparably affect the heart, the respiratory system, and the brain. In a society that neglects people with disabilities, it isn't too cynical to say that we are unlikely to provide the supports and care necessary to people who suffer from long COVID. Many families still seek answers from institutions that allowed their loved ones to die of neglect as COVID-19 swept through long-term care facilities and retirement homes. Disability rights activists are still reeling from decisions made by bureaucrats who triaged hospitalized patients based on their "pre-existing medical conditions" and life expectancy. Who gets oxygen when ventilators are in short supply, who gets life-saving antiviral medications, whose life is most precious?

COVID-19 is a disease that disproportionately ravages the poorest, most disadvantaged populations, Indigenous communities, Black people, and other people of colour in Canada and abroad. Collectively, we are responsible for at least 10.5 million children orphaned by COVID-19 worldwide.[4] Those are children who lost a parent or caregiver to COVID-19 because we failed to act, we turned our political backs globally, we "moved on." Those children are now at increased risk of poverty, abuse, mental illness, and institutionalization.

Locally, Ottawa Public Health declared that we are entering the eighth wave of COVID-19. Cases are on the rise, and hospital emergency rooms are yet again overwhelmed. Politicians refuse to allow public health units to act. The leaders of our medical associations have asserted that healthcare is in crisis in Canada, to no avail. How do we reconcile that some politicians in Ontario and across Canada assert that there are "no waves," that we have to "learn to live with" COVID-19, while public health tells us that we are entering a new wave? We are told repeatedly to brace for impact, to step up and care for our patients, yet we must also brace for the next wave of disinformation, and the next onslaught of harassment.

As a family physician, my days are spent speaking with patients who have long COVID; patients whose children are struggling to breathe as they are infected for the second, third, and fourth time; patients who are upset that they are being forced to return to workplaces where nobody will mask or isolate when sick; and patients whose family members died from COVID-19 and who are grieving at the same time as dealing with trying to keep themselves safe. Yet my colleagues and I then walk into businesses, workplaces, schools, airports, and we board buses and subways, we go to donate blood, and we are surrounded by people who say, "I don't need to mask. It isn't required. The pandemic is over." Our sense of brokenness is tied to a disappointing sense of the loss of civic responsibility. Who are we left to advocate for if the population is generally complacent, if people are fundamentally selfish, if "you're on your own" is the new normal?

It is, indeed, every person for themselves. Politicians in Canada and abroad have encouraged people to take off their masks and show off their smiles, and declared that we must normalize recurrent infections with long-term consequences, while public health units feebly encourage people to mask "when they feel it is appropriate." There are no longer travel restrictions, or vaccine mandates, or mask requirements, or requirements to isolate for people who are contagious with COVID-19. There are no protections

for people who are immunocompromised as they return
to classrooms or workplaces. Public health agencies locally and globally have advised people to make their own
"choices," a clear signal that preventative measures and the
message that "we're in this together" have been supplanted
by a focus on individualism, a mark of the impact of
anti-vaxx, anti-mask, anti-science, and anti-democracy campaigns of mis/disinformation. People are left to make their
own decisions, in the context of disinformation, about the
risks and long-term consequences of COVID-19 infection.

We feel broken, demoralized, exhausted, angry, and impa-
tient with what we perceive as the lack of caring around us.

Breaking Canadians is but a moment in time, a snapshot
of our experiences, a small piece of a complex puzzle. It
is about the fragmentation of our healthcare system, pre-
existing social inequalities, and the impact of colonialism,
racism, ableism, and ageism on the well-being of people
in Canada. We are each writing from the vantage point of
years of navigating the pandemic in our lives and in our
work. This volume spans the period from March 2020 to
October 2022. Some pieces were submitted early on in the
pandemic, some in the third wave, others in the sixth, seventh, and eighth wave.

It takes courage to speak out, to tell one's story. Some of
us have been threatened, have endured harassment and
vitriol at our offices, at our homes, by tabloids, and on social
media. Some contributors have been confronted by hostile

people in our streets and workplaces, and many have experienced schisms in their families.

Our stories are our own. These are tales about our experiences, how we cope with loss, how we survive financially, how we navigate the pandemic, and who helps and who hinders us. Some of the contributors to *Breaking Canadians* use pseudonyms to protect themselves from further harm.

As the editor of this volume, I have not fact-checked the details of people's lives. I have not paid anyone to contribute to this book, nor will I gain from its publication (all proceeds, if there are any royalties, will be donated to organizations that support vulnerable populations). Some of the writers are academics, healthcare professionals, or other professionals. Some have published or spoken publicly, some have privilege, and some have never been invited to speak. I ask you to interpret the personal narratives that are included here in the context of systemic inequalities and societal challenges.

In an effort to include as many diverse voices as possible from across Canada, I acknowledge that geography, race, language, gender, professional and educational status, disability, age, and other socio-economic barriers shape all publications, including one such as this. I was inundated with thought-provoking, heart-wrenching stories when I put out a call for submissions for *Breaking Canadians*. The stories that were excluded from this volume were no less important than those that were included.

Twitter was the primary social media platform on which I engaged in conversations with colleagues in healthcare, health research, and health communication. The *Breaking Canadians* call for submissions went out on Twitter, and from there it was shared on Facebook and elsewhere on social media, by email, and by word of mouth.

The use of social media to reach out to Canadians is, itself, a bias. Twitter is an echo chamber; we follow each other based on shared values. When I became active on Twitter, it was a space dominated by men. I made a concerted effort early on to follow thousands of women in medicine and other fields, and to selectively follow men who were allies. I described myself as a Jewish feminist, and repeatedly called out misogyny, racism, antisemitism, bigotry, and other forms of discrimination in my tweets and comments. As a result, many of the people who followed me on Twitter were people who similarly stood up for values of equity, diversity, and inclusivity. My reliance on social media to engage with Canadians is nevertheless a bias that shaped my experience of the COVID-19 pandemic, as well as ultimately the publication of this book.

Of note, a few people (including an RN) reached out who wanted to share their stories about why they believe vaccines are evil, and why they think their "freedoms" have been infringed upon. I made the decision, unapologetically, not to include their stores in *Breaking Canadians*. This book is not a vehicle for them to further spread their disinformation.

The brokenness that we describe in this volume is not uniquely Canadian. Our stories are also the product of global systems of media and technology that actively promote disinformation like wildfire.

By the time *Breaking Canadians* goes to print, thousands more people will die of COVID-19, and hundreds of thousands more will be infected. The pandemic is not over, locally or globally. Our challenge, on behalf of Canadians, is to address the brokenness of our systems, to address the chasms and barriers and failures that our predecessors created, and that our current leaders and institutions perpetuate.

Most of us who are professionals and academics contributing to this volume did not know each other prior to the COVID-19 pandemic. We came together, as community leaders in healthcare and education, to advocate for our patients and our communities. We have no personal connection to the laypeople whose stories are included in this volume. We are collectively commenting on the institutional gaps and policy failures that affect the well-being of Canadians.

As you read *Breaking Canadians*, I hope that it will help each of you feel less broken. Our shared goal is to shift the conversation and focus of responsibility to the bigger picture, to an understanding of the brokenness of the systems in which we live and work, here and globally. Systemic inequalities, ableism, ageism, and racism that existed before the pandemic will persist long after COVID-19 is a faint memory, unless we work together towards change.

When all is said and done, tomes will be written about which jurisdictions were most successful in mitigating the spread and impact of COVID-19. I leave it to others to review that data and report back. Will we pay attention to those lessons? Have politicians and public health experts, leaders in Canadian healthcare and other institutions, acknowledged and learned from their mistakes? Will we be in any way better prepared for the next pandemic? Where will members of the Canadian public and global citizens turn for health information in 2023 and beyond? Will people be wiser or more confused and distrustful? Can we take better care of each other? In short, can we fix what is broken in Canada and elsewhere?

There are more questions than there are answers. I am cynical, as a physician. I look at my patients – young and old – who are sick with their third or fourth COVID-19 infection, the patients who are suffering from long COVID, the lack of mitigation or supports, and the widespread disregard for the well-being of vulnerable populations, and I am not hopeful. Through my lens as an anthropologist, I am wary of our society's focus on individuals. I am pessimistic about political agendas that focus on consumerism and wealth. I do not hold out great hope that we will fix the brokenness in our healthcare system, so long as provinces and territories push for profit and privatization. As a Canadian citizen, I am distraught by a general lack of empathy, by people's refusal or inability to consider broad, global, long-term consequences of our (in)actions. While organized hate escalates around the world and those of us who stand up to systemic discrimination and inequalities are threatened and harassed, who will be left to speak?

Midway through the pandemic, I met Dr. Theresa Tam, the chief public health officer of Canada, in an Ottawa high school gymnasium at one of the Jabapalooza COVID-19 vaccine clinics that I ran. We only spoke briefly, as she was there for her own booster, not in a public health capacity. She looked exhausted. I was brimming with energy, fuelled by the room full of volunteers whom I'd learned I could count upon to help get done whatever was needed. "This is a marathon, not a sprint," Dr. Tam said to me. I often think about her words. We need to pace ourselves, to know when to rest. Rather than a marathon, we need to run a relay, to know that we build on the work of others who went ahead of us, and there are those behind us ready to carry on.

Moving from a sports to a music analogy, we must rely on those around us, a chorus of voices, to carry the tune, to harmonize, to riff, to give us the time and space to recover when our voices are hoarse from exhaustion, when we gasp for breath not because of the mask we are wearing but because we are shaking with fury that we have to say the same things over and over again. One voice is easy to silence. A chorus of voices is much more powerful.

So where to next?

Breaking Canadians is a testament to our commitment to persist in asking questions, and to advocate for change. Our shared challenge is to find ways to address what is broken, even when things feel quite bleak. We must work together, as the burden of this work is too much for any of us on our own.

Please take our baton, or join our chorus. Here's to standing up and speaking out, like our lives depend upon it, together.

NILI KAPLAN-MYRTH, MD, CCFP, FCFP, PHD, is a school trustee in Ottawa, a family physician with a clinic in central Ottawa, a medical anthropologist, and a mother of three children. She writes about health policy and politics, including three previous books: *Hard Yakka: Transforming Indigenous Health Policy and Politics; Women Who Care: Women's Stories of Health Care and Caring;* and *Much Madness, Divinest Sense: Women's Stories of Mental Health and Health Care.*

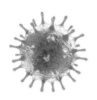

PART I

IN THE COMMUNITY

We begin this volume about the COVID-19 pandemic with the diverse voices of patients, parents, seniors, children, caregivers, people with disabilities, and other community members.

Each person tells their own story, in their own style, about how they navigated the fragmented healthcare system and overcame geographic, political, economic, and psychosocial barriers in their quest for care for themselves and their loved ones.

Although these vignettes of people's pandemic experiences are only a few small threads, when they are woven together they tell a story about our connectedness.

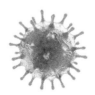

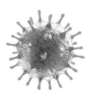

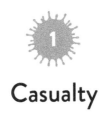

Casualty

LYNDA HURLEY

Four months into the pandemic, my husband was diagnosed with an aggressive inoperable brain tumour. I was allowed to be with him at his first appointment after he was diagnosed. He was alone after that. I sat in the hospital parking lot as he went through chemotherapy and radiation and difficult conversations. Listening on the phone in the car to a masked doctor explaining his treatment was hard to hear, both physically and emotionally. It was difficult to make any of the decisions that had to be made on an ongoing basis: decisions about changes in his chemotherapy, how those changes would best be addressed, or whether to have another MRI. I was my husband's advocate and, at this crucial time in his life, he really needed me beside him, not on a phone.

For the first nine months, he was able to have a fairly normal life. Although we knew the tumour was there, and

even though he was undergoing treatment, he was in no
pain and could participate in most of the activities he had
done before, except enjoy anything with his family because
of COVID. Pre-pandemic, we would have had time to make
memories that we could always treasure. Not to be. We had
to spend the time alone to protect his compromised immune
system.

My husband's life was always about family. Now, he was
going to die and whatever precious time he might have had
with them was being taken away. By the time he was vaccinated, he was too ill to have meaningful moments.

COVID stole my husband from his family when he
needed us the most.

Not a COVID death, not long COVID, but a COVID
casualty.

LYNDA HURLEY lives in Toronto. Her husband passed away on
21 September 2021.

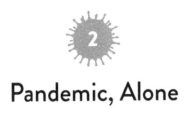

Pandemic, Alone

LEORA EISEN

For three months, all she saw was a hand. A hand would pass her lunch on a tray or put a thermometer up to her forehead. Even with her hearing aids in, the voices sounded muffled behind the masks.

My mother lived in a private retirement home. Thankfully, during that first lockdown, while many seniors' homes resembled scenes from a disaster movie, her building was quiet.

Behind closed doors, quiet can be dangerous.

As a little girl, she hid under a grand piano that belonged to her uncle's non-Jewish girlfriend. Her hearing was perfect then. She waited until the boot clicks on the cobblestones and the sharp barks of German shepherds faded away.

One day, her family was rounded up with others in the town square. Every week, Romanian police gathered Jews to send them to the trains, under the careful watch of their German superiors. Apparently, Jews were supposed to be rounded up on a particular day – say, a Tuesday. Today was Thursday. The Nazi officer gave the Romanians a tongue-lashing, and the Jews were let go. "The Germans liked order," she explained.

My siblings and I never heard this, or any of her wartime memories, until our kids interviewed her for a school project. She told them how a German governess taught her the Nazi salute behind her parents' back; how her brother was taunted and beaten on his way home from school; how her father was sent to a labour camp; how the SS commandeered her family's house; how they escaped on a ship crammed with people and sewage and survived on a diet of sardines.

"Why didn't you tell us this before?" I wondered. "We survived," she said with a shrug. "Who was I to complain? I was one of the lucky ones."

For three months, we weren't allowed to visit. At first, she kept busy reading, watching the news and playing Scrabble on her iPad. We spoke on the phone – she didn't have the tech skills or interest to master video calls.

My mother was used to looking after herself. She had come to Canada knowing no one, been widowed twice, and lost a daughter to cancer. She knew what it was like to be lonely.

But this – this was different.

My mother had Parkinson's. Without her daily exercise classes, or any meaningful human contact, she became weaker, shakier. What was supposed to be just a routine urinary tract infection sent her spiralling.

This resilient woman who spoke several languages, monitored the stock market, and played a mean game of bridge, began to lose it.

As the days blurred, so did her thoughts. Eventually, over Zoom, she was diagnosed with Alzheimer's. "It's like a perfect storm," her neurologist told me. "When you already have cognitive deficits from Parkinson's, the brain has no gas left in the tank to deal with the isolation and dementia."

Despite everything she had already lived through, she said those months of lockdown, in complete isolation, with no one to visit with or talk to, were the worst months she had ever endured.

You can't talk to a hand.

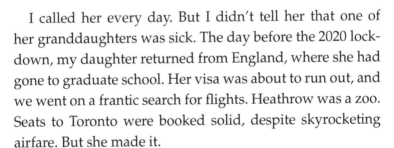

I called her every day. But I didn't tell her that one of her granddaughters was sick. The day before the 2020 lockdown, my daughter returned from England, where she had gone to graduate school. Her visa was about to run out, and we went on a frantic search for flights. Heathrow was a zoo. Seats to Toronto were booked solid, despite skyrocketing airfare. But she made it.

Within two days, her symptoms started. Fever, chills, aches, cough, exhaustion, trouble walking up the stairs. She slept on her stomach so she could breathe, unaware that this was a medical technique called "proning." My husband brought home a pulse oximeter from his locked down dental office so we'd know when her oxygen was too low. He took her to the ER twice, waiting in the parking lot while brave health workers in Hazmat suits checked her lungs. She was never tested – tests were only for the hospitalized back then – but she was "presumed" COVID-19 positive.

We did our best to stay apart from each other. But nine days after her symptoms began, mine kicked in – the weirdest symptoms I've ever experienced. It felt like a piano was sitting on my chest. Then another part of my body would tighten, as if I was in labour and having a contraction, and then my shoulder or stomach or butt would feel like I had just been punched or run a marathon. I was morbidly fascinated by what this strange virus could do to a human body.

I never told my mom.

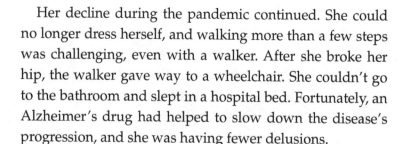

Her decline during the pandemic continued. She could no longer dress herself, and walking more than a few steps was challenging, even with a walker. After she broke her hip, the walker gave way to a wheelchair. She couldn't go to the bathroom and slept in a hospital bed. Fortunately, an Alzheimer's drug had helped to slow down the disease's progression, and she was having fewer delusions.

Her mind was sharp enough to know she was losing her dignity. She told me people who died in their sleep were lucky.

One day during lunch, she lost consciousness. A caregiver alerted the staff and then called my brother and me. The paramedics thought she might have had a seizure. Her blood pressure and oxygen levels zigzagged. But after a week of treatment and tests in the hospital, she rebounded.

The day after she returned to the retirement home, she did a yoga class in her wheelchair. The next day, she ate dinner in the dining room, treating herself to a steak.

I normally didn't visit in the evenings, but when she didn't answer my call, I went to check. It was strange – the phone line was hooked up, but there was no ringtone.

She was already tucked in bed, tired but in good spirits. We chatted. She wondered why there was a light reflected on the closet door facing her bed.

I didn't see any light. I stroked her hand, and said I love you.

The next morning, she was gone.

LEORA EISEN is a documentary filmmaker in Toronto.

Present Tense

TANIA J. SPENCER

One year after we settle in Whitehorse, the World Health Organization (WHO) declares a pandemic. At first, the virus seems faraway. But within days, it is in 192 countries. Like everyone else, we stock up on supplies, and enquire about homemade masks. It is a bad time not to know anyone in a small town.

Our sons are about to make their first funded film, ironically about grief. We are out scouting for locations. It is cold, the sun dazzling. I photograph an old mattress dumped in the snow, too deep to explore. It is my idea to grab a cappuccino downtown, and rethink the location. As people who have travelled for decades, our favourite café is full of global tourists who come up here to see the Aurora, and sometimes ride in a dog sled. On this Saturday morning, the café thrums with excitement and swishing Gore-Tex. This last outing in early March 2020 could easily be captioned "… in happier days."

A few days later, when the shortness of breath sets in, I decide to separate myself from my family. I ferret out a sleeping bag and blow-up mattress for my partner, his toothbrush, clothes. From now on he will sleep downstairs in the living room. I also put a refuse bin upstairs because nothing I touch will leave the room. Some refuse bags for my laundry. A can of Lysol, wipes, a roll of kitchen paper towels, Tylenol, and Betadine gargle. For company, a phone, laptop, a Doris Lessing memoir. And a pen and an all-weather notebook belonging to my partner, a geologist. It is mostly empty save for a few pages scrawled with words like Au deposits, Wernecke Breccia, Vein/Breccia, Skarn/replacement, Porphyry/sheeted veins …

The first note I write is the number for the local communicable disease office. I will phone this number at least three times, maybe four. I am too sick to remember.

Next, I record which symptoms, in what order. As well as fourteen strokes on a line. Each day I put a strike through one. This helps keep track of the days, which quickly blur. Beyond the room, real life continues. Zoom meetings, phone calls, tapping keys, the clink of dishes in sudsy water, vacuum cleaning, supper on the table, long teenage showers. While I keep as still as possible, anchored with painkillers. And survive on clementines, digestive biscuits, and English breakfast tea. The Doris Lessing memoir is soon abandoned.

I am in isolation, and my family, in quarantine. Colleagues drop off groceries. No one tells us to do this. The script is tight: if you haven't travelled, you cannot possibly have COVID-19. I will later meet others also told they don't meet the criteria for testing. They will also have symptoms consistent with COVID-19. Also be as sick as they have never before been.

I learn how to ask for help on the communicable disease line, when it's not enough to say I can't breathe. The nurse is firm. You don't meet the criteria. I back up. Okay. These are stressful times for all of us. And for you too. I understand that. It's still no, the nurse says.

The last time I call my voice won't sound like my own. It will have holes in it like a net, the timbre stringy. You've probably just got a bad flu, I'm told.

In the early days of the pandemic, a positive PCR test is the gatekeeper to medical care for COVID-19. Yukoners with symptoms are instructed not to go to the ER, the walk-in clinic, or pharmacies. Instead, they should phone their family doctor. I do not have a family doctor, and phoning is getting me nowhere.

The only thing to do is be calmer than everybody else. I email five high-profile office-bearers in town. I explain that I can't breathe and can't get help. What should I do? No one replies. I email the hospital. Six days later a response: "I'm sorry I didn't see this sooner."

By now I am gasping. My hands and lips are cyanotic. I go to the ER.

The first thing the triage nurse notices are my hands. Are they normally that colour? No. She stands up, and reaches for a mask. At that point, I have no idea how much I will revisit this moment in the years to come. The gratitude I will feel for this nurse.

The doctor asks if I've travelled. No. After some routine tests (but no PCR test), he says I can go home. And, no, he isn't going to consider COVID because "it isn't in the Yukon yet."

I go home, back to isolation even though I don't have to. Because, according to the doctor, I'm not sick. For days, my heart mashes against my ribs like a fish trying to get back to water. Two days later, the Yukon confirms its first two official cases.

A week later, still struggling to breathe, still with blue hands and lips, I am back in the ER. Although the hospital is empty, it is braced. A different triage nurse observes my elevated heart rate and asks if I am "nervous." No. I just can't breathe.

This time I get a PCR test but am told not to come back as the hospital is going to become a "very dangerous" place. I avoid the ER for the next two years.

It takes thirteen days to get the result, which is negative. That must be why nobody phoned. I have been tested too late, and now there is proof that I do not have COVID-19.

On day fifteen, I finish my isolation. Within a week my family has the same symptoms. This time we look after ourselves. There's no begging for a PCR test, no phoning anyone, no going to the ER. After a week, my partner and sons mostly recover, but I develop long COVID before the name is even coined.

There is no word to describe what I have. Many nights, I push myself up on my fists, my mouth wide open. Every sixth gasp or so, small relief. As someone else describes it, you open your mouth and nothing happens.

I seem to have forgotten how to breathe. Up on my pillows, I hunch around the possibility of breath. And what rhymes with it. I have the vascular, neurological, multi-organ version of COVID-19. It doesn't show up in chest X-rays or blood tests. My hands are purple for two years. And swollen. I have to have my rings resized. Equally hard to believe – that even supine, my heart can hit 250 beats per minute. I also lose handfuls of hair and develop bruising without cause.

And I don't need a brain scan to know that my brain is injured. For two years, I wake up feeling concussed. My dreams are evanescent. My life feathered with Post-it Notes. I lose my short-term memory, vocabulary, imagination, spark, patience, and joy. In their stead, I have post-traumatic stress disorder.

I can't process numbers. I forget how to spell "doughnut." Prepositions are a puzzle. I mangle idioms. And although I once lived in the Middle East, I can't remember if it is a compound word. I read one book twice, obliviously enjoying it both times.

And although I am a photographer, I struggle to read some 2D images. In a photo of a piebald calf, there is a lag before I integrate areas of light and dark into one animal.

I have hallucinations, olfactory and other. One day, I recognize people I know I don't know. Sometimes a buzzer goes off in my head that no one else can hear. And I hallucinate that one of our sons can't breathe. At 3 a.m., I am at their doors wanting to know who. The geologist giggles, and he's not a giggler.

When we go for walks in the forest, my family waits for me because I cannot breathe properly. Sometimes I feign interest in animal tracks, or fiddle with my gloves.

In that first year of the pandemic, two women are found floating in bodies of water in the Yukon. I think of them more than I should. Because if you can't breathe, nothing matters.

The virus has taken a cricket bat to my life, leaving everything out of register, the colours knocked apart. For the first year, I have a grocery list of about fifty different symptoms and no medical care. I self-medicate with supplements I have to google. I have no idea what helps, if anything at all.

The backbone of my self-medication, however, is something with even less medical basis: books about swimming, every and all kinds.

I read James Nestor's book *Deep* about freediving. In 1894, a French physiologist called Charles Richet did some horrible things to ducks to test the effect water has on the vagus nerve. He showed that ducks lived longer underwater because of an oxygen conserving reflex that slowed the heart rate via the vagus nerve. He thought the same might apply to humans. And in 1962, a physiologist named Per Scholander proves him right and names the effect of cold water on the human body the Master Switch of Life (aka the "mammalian dive reflex").

With this in mind, throughout a Yukon winter, I take two cold showers a day to try to reset my nervous system. I also drink lurid smoothies to increase my nitric oxide. As for Nietzsche's wry observation – "Everyone who has ever built anywhere a new heaven first found the power thereto in his own hell" – most probably.

A year later, in 2021, I am allocated a family doctor, tested for everything I don't have (in the beginning, long COVID is a diagnosis of exclusion), and am prescribed an inhaler that underestimates the condition.

Unlike many others now living with long COVID, I begin my fourth year much recovered, but certain of nothing. Numerous studies show how SARS-CoV-2 assaults the brain, and I have also recently developed atrial fibrillation – a direct function of long COVID. Whatever the future may bring, I live gratefully in the present.

TANIA J. SPENCER lives in Whitehorse, Yukon. She is a writer and photographer. Her photographic work has been exhibited in numerous locations, including Iqaluit, the Northwest Territories, and South Africa. Her writing has been published in journals, books, and newspapers.

A Community Divided

ANONYMOUS

I live in a tranquil farming community in the heart of the "Bible Belt" of rural southern Ontario. Like most people everywhere, residents of my town are typically industrious, caring, and friendly. There are many different religious groups in my community, and prior to the pandemic, they usually co-existed peacefully. I never really expected that my town would be the subject of national news stories – until the pandemic disrupted our lives and divided us.

COVID's sudden arrival sparked panic and fear, as people listened to the media for updates and guidance. Out of a sense of community responsibility, most of us were willing to follow public health guidelines. We listened carefully to messaging about the importance of handwashing and staying home as much as possible to stop the spread. We watched heartbreaking stories about healthcare workers battling COVID-19 on the front lines in hospitals. Whenever

I ventured out, streets were eerily quiet, and patrolled by police cars to ensure compliance with the new social distancing rules. It was unsettling.

Some of us wore masks when we left home for essential reasons, and we supported local businesses as much as we could. Others perceived COVID-19 to be an urban problem, confidently proclaiming, "There's no COVID here," as if we were somehow exempt from what was happening everywhere else. I remember seeing a few unmasked acquaintances chatting in close proximity in a store. They were blaming masked protestors at the outdoor Black Lives Matter demonstrations for amplifying the pandemic, with no sense of irony. I did not share their views. Clearly, we needed better messaging about how COVID-19 spreads through the air, from one human being to another, as we breathe and speak. It was no wonder that our town became a COVID-19 hotspot.

One local group had a particularly divisive effect on our community. It was the now-infamous Church of God Restoration (COGR). The firebrand leader of the COGR, Pastor Henry Hildebrandt, encouraged his followers to oppose all public health measures. He spread conspiracy theories about the "evils" of medicine, vaccinations, and government regulations. People with no church affiliation began to follow him for his political views. He organized a so-called freedom rally that brought a large crowd into our downtown, shutting down local businesses. Our mayor – who declared a state of emergency in response to the potential for violence at the rally – was targeted with threats. The media flocked to town to cover the rallies, and we developed an unfortunate reputation as an anti-masking and anti-vaccination community. The conflict deepened between people who opposed public health measures for personal "freedom" and people who recognized the need for public health measures. Our town was avoided.

Unlike other faith groups who complied with public health guidance,[1] the COGR continued to hold large indoor church gatherings that flouted provincial restrictions until a court ordered the police to lock the doors of the church. The congregation defied the court orders with large, unmasked services in the parking lot each Sunday. Some members were charged for being physically aggressive towards the police officers and also towards the editor of a local newspaper who filmed the incident. The pastor's son, Herbert Hildebrandt, was also charged with assaulting an elderly man for putting up a pro-masking sign on the public road allowance along the highway.

Local residents who supported public health measures lined the highway near the church in their vehicles to show their opposition to the unlawful gatherings.

COVID broke our community. Maskless people forced their way into local businesses. Some wore T-shirts emblazoned with slogans such as "Faith Not Fear," or wore a hoodie to hide their faces. For the people who owned and worked in these stores, their presence was terrifying. The two grocery stores had to hire security guards to keep the peace.

The COGR launched a motion to challenge any restrictions on its large indoor gatherings in court, claiming that any limitation whatsoever on their religious freedoms violated their Charter rights.[2] It lost. The judge ruled that freedoms are not absolute and need to be balanced with the competing rights of others. This is an important message for all Canadians. Your rights end where the rights of others begin.

I believe that the people who were flouting public health regulations may not have had the insight to express their needs more constructively. Church members seemed to be indoctrinated with messaging that appeared to allow an authoritarian leader to exert coercive control over their lives, and caused them to act in ways that I found surprising.[3] Unfortunately, their actions were putting the larger community at risk of infection and severe health outcomes. This lack of concern for public well-being is precisely why we need laws that limit the potential for harm when people act without regard for consequences.

I have mixed feelings towards my community. The sense of security that I felt living here has been shaken. I am deeply disappointed by the intolerance, violence, and lack of consideration for the well-being of fellow community members that some residents displayed.

As members of society, we have a moral responsibility to protect the well-being of others. Social cohesion makes us stronger. And if we don't respect each other, if we cannot be tolerant towards people who have different opinions, our communities will remain divided long after this pandemic is over.

The author of this piece has chosen to remain anonymous.

BC – Breaking Cancer

DR. JAIGRIS HODSON

The healthcare system in British Columbia was breaking before COVID-19 started. Years of cuts and consolidation had left the majority of people (70 per cent, in fact) in my city without a family doctor.[1] Despite the stress of the pandemic, burned-out healthcare workers managed to keep the system functioning – if only barely, according to the organization Protect Our Province BC.[2] Unfortunately for me, my breast cancer diagnosis occurred in 2021, during the height of the COVID-19 pandemic when I learned first-hand that the healthcare system was truly broken.

If the healthcare system hadn't been so broken, a doctor might have found my cancer before COVID-19. By the time I found it myself, it had progressed to Stage 3. I had been living in BC for years without access to a primary physician. I had no annual check-ups, no recommendation to get a yearly mammogram after age forty, and no idea that I even should be worried about cancer at the age of forty-two. As a result of COVID-19, many of my medical appointments were by Telehealth, which was ineffective in making a proper diagnosis.

The healthcare system in British Columbia is broken.

I expected the BC Cancer health service to be spared from COVID-19. BC Cancer seemed to be separate from the issues we were hearing about in the news, like full ICUs or limited access to ventilators. But it was not. Despite being diagnosed at the end of June, my treatment did not start until the middle of August. Treatment delays for my cancer increased the likelihood of premature death. I had to go into my treatments alone, with no support person as I had toxic but necessary chemotherapy.

Pre-pandemic, people said that the care at BC Cancer was great. I wasn't able to experience that care. I couldn't get to know my kind and competent chemo nurses because they were constantly run off their feet, and I never saw the same nurse twice. I could not follow up on important genetic test results that revealed I possessed a mutation that should influence the course of my care. I almost ended up getting the wrong surgery – a single mastectomy, rather than the double mastectomy that was recommended.

The healthcare system in British Columbia is broken.

My oncologist must have burned out: he left his practice. I got a letter from BC Cancer telling me that parking had changed, but no communication that my oncologist had changed. From November until March, I had no oncologist and no one to explain the results of my surgery. My chemo nurse let me know that my oncologist had left. I think she assumed that I knew. On one visit, she looked at my chart and said, "Oh, Dr. So-and-So – he's leaving," and by the time I could follow up on this piece of information, he had already gone.

The healthcare system in British Columbia is broken.

An ice-cold fear paralyzed me. Between finishing chemo in December 2021 and my scheduled surgery in late January 2022, the BC minister of health kept repeating that surgeries were being cancelled due to the fifth wave of COVID-19.

Entering what is now a sixth wave, I'm paralyzed with a different kind of fear. The immune suppression that occurs as a result of chemotherapy can last up to a year, and yet there are no protections to stop the spread of COVID-19. As an immune-compromised person, I'm told I need to protect myself, but I have no data to judge the risk levels in my community. I am essentially under house arrest watching everyone else "return to normal" – as if such disregard for vulnerable or at-risk people ought to be normal. What I wish BC Health could do is more clearly communicate to BC residents about how to protect themselves and each other with non-pharmaceutical interventions like masks, far-UV, and ventilation. I wish I could have the information I need about COVID-19 levels in my community so I could better protect myself. I wish that guidelines for N95 mask wearing in hospitals could change. Finally, I wish that money in the system could be diverted from managers and bureaucrats to fund more front-line doctors and nurses. These changes are all possible, and I wonder why there seems to be no interest in making them.

The healthcare system in British Columbia is broken.

And now it is breaking me. As more physicians and nurses leave their practice, as lines and wait times get longer for diagnosis, treatment, and medical testing, and as more and more people present with complex health issues due to long COVID, I wonder if I will survive. After surgery, chemotherapy, and radiation, my cancer is at bay – for now. But without the healthcare infrastructure we need, I despair about what could happen if it ever comes back.

JAIGRIS HODSON is the Canada Research Chair (tier 2) in Digital Communication for the Public Interest. Her SSHRC and CIHR funded research examines such interdisciplinary topics as online harassment, misinformation, and science and health communication. In 2021, during the height of the COVID-19 pandemic, Hodson was diagnosed with breast cancer. Since then, she has pivoted her research focus to understanding how young people use digital tools during and following a cancer diagnosis.

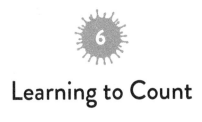

Learning to Count

ELEANOR RAMPHAL

Whenever I teach about an event in which people died, I ask students to first create a tally of every life lost. The last time I did this exercise, we were discussing Canada's residential schools. I told students I was asking them to do this because, if it were my child, I would want every discussion about residential schools to acknowledge her, even if it was just a mark of chalk on the board. It is important to make those lives visible. As I write this on 21 April 2022, 38,696 Canadians have died from COVID-19.[1] That number isn't real for me yet. We haven't done a tally.

I'm a teacher in Quebec, and I don't want COVID. I don't think that's too much to ask of a preventable disease. Yet everywhere I go, people are ready to infect me. Few really enforce mask mandates in school, or the two metres people must keep from each other – sorry, one metre as of last month. A colleague happily announced she got COVID last week as we began our in-person meeting today. She's past the five-day mark, but below the ten-day one, which means she still has to wear a mask, according to the current rules. She didn't, even though I kind of, sort of, said, "Don't you still have to wear a mask for a few more days? I think that's a thing." She laughed it off. As mask mandates crumbled, I upped my own mask game. I still wear a mask at home after every major known COVID exposure at work to avoid infecting my family. I've had another week of eating outside, showering when my family's not at home, sleeping with a towel shoved under the door and a HEPA filter blasting next to the bed.

But COVID may not get me at work. It will probably arrive when my daughter brings it home from school. Lunch hour in her school is not safe. Schools don't mandate open windows or that students eat outside when the weather is nice – probably because saying it's safer to eat outside in May implies that it's unsafe to eat indoors in January, and schools don't want that message circulating. I know of one parent who asked a school to share with the other families in her child's class that her son just tested positive. The school refused. Schools won't do anything they haven't been ordered to do by the government. The only thing schools are doing, in fact, is something they have never done before – refusing donations. My request to donate a HEPA filter to my then-unvaccinated daughter's class went up through the chain of command as they tried to figure out how to say no. A few days later, the principal informed me that the school ventilation systems "comply with ministerial requirements." Thinking this was a question of equity,

I offered to donate one to all the classes in her grade. No again. But don't worry – I was assured that students sanitize their hands throughout the day, as though we hadn't been inundated with evidence that COVID is airborne.

I teach over 150 children, and I feel sick when I think about how many have likely had COVID. It's horrifying given all we know about the long-term damage COVID inflicts on the brain, blood, and lungs.[2] I don't want the guilt of having transmission occur in my class. I try to keep windows open, remembering that my job is first to keep children safe, and second to teach them something.

I hope that after all this, we work to make schools safer. Ideally, schools will open windows whenever they can. We will have legislation that entitles us to clean air, to a CO_2 reading well under 1,000 parts per million. People will wear respirators in public spaces, especially where there are children who cannot consent to a risk to their health. Children will get COVID once a decade instead of once a year.

For today, we need to grapple with these questions (raise your hand if you know the answers): Why have we forgotten our children? Who needs to be held accountable? When will we teach about the great COVID tragedy and tally the deaths on a chalkboard?

ELEANOR RAMPHAL comes from a family full of teachers. It's a job that's never boring, they said. After six years, she has to agree.

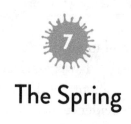

The Spring

DR. DAVID KEEGAN

Waterborne Outbreak

It was around 1999 when I was working on the coast of Newfoundland that I got entangled in my first significant infectious disease outbreak. I was a rural family doctor for a region of 13,500 people: clinics, emergency, inpatient care, palliative care, long-term care – the list goes on. I loved my work, the people I worked with, and those I cared for. On that particular day, I had cared for two people with salmonella and one with giardia ("beaver fever"). All three were quite unwell with one or two needing to be hospitalized.

Whenever you hear of bacterial or parasitic intestinal disease as a doctor, you immediately try to identify the source so you can prevent more people from getting sick. On the phone with public health the day the lab reports came back, I shared my suspicion: The Spring.

The Spring was a natural spring on the side of the highway. I had heard about it many, many times in my training and practice in this community. "The town water is no good." "The Spring water is the best water possible." There was some truth about the town water. It had a brownish tinge. This was later determined to be from trihalomethanes (THMs), created when the then only moderately filtered water's organic materials came in contact with chlorine. The THM level was later proven to be linked with higher rates of cancer.

Public health investigated my concern and, sure enough, The Spring's water was filled with multiple different disease-causing organisms, including salmonella and giardia. Some people were pleased when a sign was placed, warning people of the dangers of drinking this contaminated water. I was surprised by the people who angrily denounced this discovery and continued to swear by the quality of this water source. A small number of my patients left my practice as my role in identifying the problem had become widely known.

I struggled to understand this reaction. If The Spring was proven to be contaminated and unsafe, the only logical response was to boil and filter it before drinking or, better yet, avoid it altogether. For some people, their emotional connection to The Spring trumped science.

2003 SARS Outbreak

The first Severe Acute Respiratory Syndrome Coronavirus (SARS-CoV-1 or SARS) epidemic hit Toronto in 2003. Early days were full of uncertainty and adrenaline. Yet there was clear communication from the provincial government that the right things would be done to control this SARS outbreak and eliminate it.

I had been working as an emergency doctor in London, Ontario, and received N95 masks and later full hazmat suits to use when caring for a person with suspected or known SARS. I was very grateful for this personal protective equipment as the virus had a 30 per cent fatality rate.

I also worked in the new Patient Transfer Authorization Centre (PTAC). It had been set up to strictly monitor and control where patients went, as a way of locking down risk of further SARS transmission. Created out of thin air and housed at the headquarters for Toronto's Emergency Medicine Services (EMS), we had to build our protocols on the fly. Still, the fact that PTAC had been set up at all was incredibly reassuring: the government was serious about doing what needed to be done. The reason seemed obvious: a choice to *not* get SARS under control would result in profound disease, death, and economic devastation.

Within six months of the first case, SARS was extinguished in Ontario: 375 Ontarians had become ill with SARS, including the forty-four who died.[1] I remember at the time a persistent vigilance extending well past the point when it seemed there were no new SARS cases. There was no fatalism. There was no minimizing. There was only the clear recognition that together we had to defeat SARS. And we did.

SARS-2 (COVID-19) Pandemic

In January 2020, word of a highly contagious virus began to spread around the globe. By March 2020, the virus itself had clearly arrived in Canada. Initially, we came together as a society, and the first wave ultimately didn't reach the astronomical number of cases and deaths as had been anticipated. Still, by 7 July 2020, over 100,000 Canadians had become ill with SARS-2 (COVID-19), of whom over 9,000 had died. These figures likely under-represent the true numbers as initially SARS-2 testing was restricted to known contacts or persons returning from other countries.

It is obvious to all that SARS-2 has been managed differently than SARS-1 (the 2003 outbreak in Toronto). For SARS-1, there had been an immediate precaution to treat it as airborne and universal airborne precautions were implemented. All healthcare workers received N95 masks. For SARS-2, however, there were early and vigorous reassurances that masks had no role in stopping the spread, even though some scientists from around the globe suggested that out of precaution we should be managing SARS-2 as if it could be airborne. Indeed, some of the reports of spreading within apartment buildings suggested it likely *was* airborne.

By the fall of 2020, there were increasing concerns that SARS-2 could be airborne, yet its airborne nature continued to be rejected by many public health officials. At the same time, the prospect of effective vaccines was growing. As vaccines became available in the first half of 2021, many governments in Canada emphasized that vaccines were the main way out of the pandemic. On 26 May 2021, Alberta premier Jason Kenney announced the rapid dismantling of most public health protections, anticipating the "best Alberta summer ever," despite only 70 per cent of Albertans having received their first dose of vaccine at the time. It seemed obvious that, with new daily SARS-2 case counts in Canada still exceeding 2,500 by the end of May 2021, it was simply premature to declare victory and remove public health protections.[2]

In other words, we needed a vaccine-plus strategy: widespread use of vaccines PLUS non-medication measures to prevent spread.

Despite Canada having been a key site for SARS-1 and having learned the value of persistent vigilance and public health protections in eradicating the virus in 2003, most Canadian provinces elected to discard this experience and rapidly dismantled protections. What had changed between SARS-1 and SARS-2?

While the government and medical community were onside for SARS-1, they were clearly at odds for SARS-2. The bravado from some politicians and public health officials in our ongoing SARS-2 pandemic reminds me of the people who still wanted to drink from The Spring despite its proven contamination. A key difference is that while all the officials and politicians recognized The Spring had, unfortunately, been proven to be dangerous, with SARS-2, numerous elected and appointed leaders have chosen to deny the science demonstrating the need for airborne measures and precautionary public health protections.

Over the last two and a half years, we have seen decision after decision been made at the expense of the health and safety of our population: the abandonment of vaccine-passports, the abandonment of mask mandates in schools, the decision to remove requirements for people with active SARS-2 to isolate, and then more broadly the failure to act in any way that recognizes the proven science that SARS-2 is airborne.[3] These decisions appear to have fuelled subsequent waves of SARS-2. Indeed, by early 2023, we were at a point where the waves of different SARS-2 variants were merging into each other and we were seeing constant circulation of the virus throughout our communities.

Importantly, we also know that the early ("acute") infection with SARS-2 is not its only harm; SARS-2 symptoms can linger causing disability (known as long COVD), the virus appears to be damaging our immune systems well after infection, leading to increased severity of other infectious diseases, and the virus massively increases the risk of a host of other conditions, including heart attack and stroke.

We learned from SARS-1 that the coronavirus behaves in largely predicable ways: it will not vanish on its own; mandatory health protections will eliminate the virus; and we can't drop health protections at the first signs they are working – they must be kept in place until it is crystal clear that viral outbreaks have been eliminated.

We are seeing mounting numbers of post-SARS-2 chronic health conditions as a result of each wave.[4] Each person's risk of disability is compounded with each successive COVID-19 infection.[5] So, why are these lessons being ignored by so many politicians and public health leaders? Why are they watching as this disaster unfolds?

I don't have any certain answers, but I can think of some possibilities.

Maybe they have such faith in vaccines that they can't comprehend the need for any other measures. Those in public health should remember that we do a number of things besides vaccinations to prevent and treat other infectious diseases and, therefore, should be able to embrace the reality that we need a "vaccine-plus" strategy.

Maybe they are worried that because they removed measures, they will be looked upon as weak or indecisive if they bring any protective measures back now. I suppose this is understandable and yet leaders are supposed to be open to new information and make decisions that protect the people they lead. In the future (and in this very book), the disastrous outcome of not acting with caution during this pandemic will be visible for all to see: massive numbers of dead and disabled Canadians. If I were a politician, I would far prefer to change direction now and be called weak than to fail to act and damage lives.

Maybe they have made a false equivalence between people and the economy, and feel that it is critical to have loosened protective measures to boost the economy. If so, this is incredibly short-sighted given the economic damage resulting from 15 per cent of the population ending up with disabling symptoms of long COVID,[6] and SARS-2 infections increasing rates of other complex and potentially disabling diseases, including heart failure, blood clots, diabetes, and stroke, by 20 per cent or more.[7] The combination of long COVID and increased disease rates caused by SARS-2 would result in massive labour shortages and likely unsustainable publicly funded services of health and income support. More importantly, if this *was* the reason for pulling back preventive health measures, it would mean leaders *knowingly* decided to sacrifice lives and health to spur economic activity. In such a case, they would have been warned that reducing preventive measures would kill and injure Canadians and yet did it anyways.

SARS-2 is not slowing down. More people died from SARS-2 in 2022 than in 2021 or 2020. Long COVID, immune dysregulation, and chronic diseases triggered by SARS-2 are mounting.

If these trends continue, we will soon be in a place where a massive proportion of our population is disabled and unable to work. We need leaders who will choose long-term public health over whatever short-term pressures have led to such poor choices. We need political and public health leaders who will stare down anti-life protestors and those seeking to discard fellow humans in order to serve the economy. Otherwise, our society will be plunged into decades of illness and despair, with a stagnant economy and a chronically overwhelmed health system.

We have to learn from our own Canadian experience with SARS-1 and focus our efforts on eradicating SARS-2 through a vaccine-plus strategy.

Just like I could not afford to pretend it was okay to drink from The Spring once we knew it was the source of terrible disease, we can't ignore that SARS-2 is airborne. We need to act to save lives and prevent disability.

DAVID KEEGAN is a family doctor and professor of family medicine in the Cumming School of Medicine at the University of Calgary. He is the founding editor of LearnFM/ApprenezMF, the collaborative Canadian family medicine curriculum for medical students (learnfm.ca). He's also a practice goalie for his kids' hockey teams.

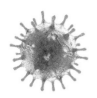

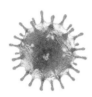

PART II

AT THE MARGINS

Breaking Canadians *is our response to a brokenness that exists outside of us. The inequities we witnessed and moral injuries that we experienced between March 2020 and October 2022 stem from a healthcare system that was already fragmented, dysfunctional, and fundamentally flawed before the COVID-19 pandemic began.*

In this section, we discuss marginalized and vulnerable populations, social injustices, biases within medical institutions, political decisions about who's invited to decision-making tables, systemic ageism, misogyny, racism, and ableism, which are key issues that played out at every level of the pandemic, with catastrophic consequences.

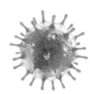

Long-Term Care or Long-Term Crime?

DR. VIVIAN STAMATOPOULOS

For a country that takes great pride in its public healthcare, we showed the world how to fail seniors and persons with disabilities living in long-term care (LTC) facilities during the COVID-19 pandemic. Truthfully, we failed them well before, but what happened over the last three years constitutes what many call Canada's "national shame."[1] Canadian LTC residents represented 81 per cent of the national reported COVID-19 deaths, compared to an average of just 38 per cent for all member countries of the Organisation for Economic Co-operation and Development (OECD).[2] Things were so bad that the Canadian Armed Forces (CAF) were deployed to some of the hardest-hit facilities in Ontario. The observation reports from their time spent inside these facilities would rock the nation. Indeed, they prompted an immediate national address by Prime Minister Justin Trudeau who would go on to promise national reform and even criminal charges for operators who were shown to fail these residents so egregiously.[3] This watershed moment came in late May 2020, just two months after the global pandemic was officially declared by the World Health Organization (WHO). In but two months, Canadians were given a painful preview of how bad things could get for residents living in LTC homes.

The Warning Signs That Something Bad Was to Come

In mid-February 2020, international news reports from Italy began circulating about the "silent surge in fatalities in nursing homes."[4] Described as "besieged castles," nursing and retirement home facilities foreshadowed what was to happen in Canada, with the virus ripping its way through the majority of private facilities that were abandoned by staff who were leaving to work in hospitals where the pay and standards of care were better.[5] Those who remained to care for the residents in nursing homes did so in incredibly trying circumstances, suffering from fatigue, disappointment, and demotivation. Widespread visitation restrictions meant that residents were often left alone in their rooms with only tablet devices to connect them with their loved ones on the outside. The attempt to replace direct contact with family with virtual visitation had limited effectiveness, especially on residents with dementia, who needed a hug, a massage, and a nearby voice.[6] Public health initiatives gave little attention to nursing homes, despite housing some of the most vulnerable populations for severe COVID-19 outcomes.[7] Personal protective equipment (PPE) and human staffing resources were diverted to hospitals while a "silent massacre"[8] unfolded in Italy's nursing homes where most COVID-19 deaths were occurring. Sound familiar?

We were warned about how bad it could get, and we could have better safeguarded the sector in the early months of the pandemic. Even without the Italian preview, we knew that older adults living in nursing homes would be especially vulnerable in a pandemic due to their advanced age and higher prevalence of chronic disease and disability. We also knew that LTC homes were historically prone to higher levels of seasonal flu and other respiratory pathogens,[9] often connected to the overall frailty of residents and the higher prevalence of shared rooms.[10] The writing was on the wall.

The first outbreak in an LTC home in Canada was declared at Lynn Valley Care Centre in British Columbia on Thursday, 5 March 2020.[11] In Ontario, the first case appeared in an LTC home on 17 March 2020.[12] Around the same time, congregate care living facilities, including LTC homes, began locking down and families were shut out. These facilities effectively became closed prisons overnight.

My Foray into Public Advocacy

I am often asked why I became a public advocate for LTC residents. Like most advocates, my own lived experiences prompted my advocacy. Just days before the first documented case of COVID-19 arrived in Canada, my grandmother passed away. She had lived in an Ontario LTC home for the better part of the previous year and, while losing someone you love is always difficult, her death forever changed me. To be sure, I have always had a soft spot in my heart for older adults, probably because of my close relationship with my grandparents. My own doctoral studies were motivated by my experiences helping to care for them as a young adult, which involved moving into their condominium as their health began to decline. Despite trying as hard as I could to keep my grandmother in her own home, her mobility began to decline, which led to falls and injuries. She eventually went on to require round-the-clock care and, before I knew it, I was told by a community care caseworker that her situation was a "crisis" and we needed to put her in LTC. No other option was given. That was the beginning of the end. Nine months later, she was gone, and I was trying to put the pieces together surrounding her death, which culminated in the securing of legal representation and, undoubtedly, the worst experience of my life.

Foreshadowing my own experiences that were to come a decade later, my first exposure to the world of LTC came through my doctoral studies when I was a research assistant to Dr. Pat Armstrong's "Re-Imagining Long-Term Residential Care" study. Dr. Armstrong is a national expert on LTC. Spanning several countries and including an international team of twenty-six researchers and fifty plus graduate students, I spent my time on the project contributing to a scan of nursing home standards and staffing levels in six countries, including Canada.[13] Even back then, I remember being surprised as to how little standardization there was in our own country to ensure LTC residents received sufficient and appropriate levels of care. That said, all the words on paper that I contributed to existed in mere black and white, until my lived experience brought them into full colour.

So here I was in late January 2020, trying to understand what happened to my grandmother and managing my grief when the news about a new infectious disease began circulating. In a few short weeks, the world as we knew it would come to a halt. One by one, cities and provinces across Canada would declare states of emergency and general lockdowns would emerge. Around this time, in the first months of the pandemic, my advocacy began, motivated single-handedly by the crude categorization of families as non-essential visitors to LTC facilities and the locking down of these facilities to the public. Heck, I knew first-hand how important families were in supporting the health and well-being of LTC residents after having spent the better part of a year inside one such facility. I also knew that keeping family caregivers out would spell disaster for the mostly female and racialized front-line workers who were chronically underpaid, understaffed, and unsupported, and who relied on extended families for much-needed extra hands in the care of the residents.

To be fair, not much was known about the virus and its transmissibility in the early days, and it is understandable why fear-based decisions would emerge at the outset. At first, I waited patiently alongside LTC families for policies to be drafted that would allow them back into the facilities. Days turned into weeks and weeks turned into months and yet nothing was happening. Story after story emerged of residents dying alone without their family present and my anger at the injustice of it grew. It was just plain wrong. However well-intentioned blanket visitation bans may have been at the beginning of the COVID-19 pandemic, they were out of touch with workers' and residents' needs. Bottom line, the bans caused clear emotional and physical distress that would result in the shocking reality of high numbers of LTC residents dying alone under this "new normal" of isolation.[14] I had no intention of quietly accepting this proposition and, about a month into the pandemic, my advocacy kicked into overdrive.

I began compiling what was happening in the news related to COVID-19 and LTC homes into what is now a master document spanning hundreds of pages. The researcher in me knew I had to organize what I was seeing and hearing to approach this methodically. Initially, my goals were twofold. First, I wanted to get as much information out to the LTC community given so little was being provided by public officials and the LTC homes themselves. I hoped this information, most of which was shared on Twitter, could equip families and workers with tips to directly advocate for better care within their own LTC homes. Second, I was determined to get families back into these facilities. To this end, I began writing about how these blanket visitation bans were not only cruel and unethical but also unlawful based on existing legislation in my province.[15] My advocacy on this issue drew the attention of NDP MPP Lisa Gretzky, with whom I would soon collaborate to draft proposed legislation that would secure the right for caregivers to have uninterrupted access to their loved ones in LTC homes and other congregate care settings via Bill 203: The More Than A

Visitor Act.[16] I spoke to as many people who would listen, including the media, politicians, and other interested stakeholders such as Ontario's Patient Ombudsman and the Ontario LTC Commissioners about the need to amend existing policies to safely reintroduce families into LTC homes and other congregate care living facilities.

As time unfolded, I would criticize problematic pandemic policies that emerged, including the disproportionate allocation of resources to acute care when LTC homes were clearly hit the hardest, and the ongoing staffing challenges.[17] I criticized anything and everything that stood out as potentially dangerous to the residents and the workers who cared for them, often focusing on Ontario. It was not long before families from across Canada began reaching out to me to share what was happening in their loved ones' LTC homes, followed by front-line staff who wished to blow the whistle on what they were seeing but could not speak out publicly for fear of reprisals. With their permission, I posted their stories to my Twitter account, often anonymously and for good reason. Keep in mind, families fear speaking out about problematic care in LTC homes during the best of times, but in an era where they were suddenly kept away from their loved ones, that fear skyrocketed. Would speaking up lead to retribution? Would it further compromise the care provided to their loved ones to whom they had no access? For staff, the obvious concern was losing their jobs or being reprimanded for drawing attention to what was happening inside the facilities. I took care to post their stories in as much detail as possible while also protecting their identities. The social media posts began to attract public attention

and, behind the scenes, I was working to connect journalists from across Canada with the families and workers who
were willing to go public.

It was not until May 2020 that I was asked to step up from
behind the scenes and provide my own commentary as an
expert/advocate. I still remember how incredibly nervous
I was preparing for those initial televised interviews, often putting in hours of research and preparation for what
would generally be condensed down to two-minute clips.
I am sure it sounds ridiculous, but I felt a deep sense of responsibility to present as accurate and reliable information
as possible. I also felt immense pressure to adequately con-
vey the gravity of the situation unfolding. The families and
workers deserved as much.

Military Reports

Tuesday, the 26th of May 2020, is a day that I will never
forget. It was the day the initial observation reports from
members of the Canadian Armed Forces deployed to five
hard-hit Ontarian LTC homes were released by media outlets. The news spread far and fast. You could not turn on a
radio or television station without hearing of the "horrors"
of Ontario's long-term care homes.[18] Fifteen pages of initial
observations for a two-week period highlighted shocking
discoveries in areas ranging from infection control to standards of practice and quality of care to staffing. Initially cov-
ering five Ontarian LTC homes, two more would be added
for a total of seven. Six of the seven, or 85 per cent, were

private, for-profit LTC homes. Although I urge everyone to read the full report, below are some highlights:[19]

1. Eatonville Care Centre: Etobicoke, Ontario (for-profit facility)

- Physicians not present in person, only accessible by phone;
- Key supplies under lock and key, not accessible by those who need them for work;
- Gross non-adherence to orders, such as regular checking of vital signs or patient turning;
- Reports of inaccurate charting;
- Inaccurate information provided to families regarding resident's status;
- Severe understaffing;
- Residents sedated with narcotics or benzodiazepines "when they are likely just sad or depressed";
- Aggressive, "abusive/inappropriate" behaviour by staff.

2. Hawthorne Place: North York, Ontario (for-profit facility)

- Major concerns regarding standards of care, including charting, and narcotics misuse;
- Food/Feeding Issues: PSWs rushed and leaving food on tables but patients could not reach the tables and/or feed themselves (therefore missing meals or going hours without eating);
- Forceful feeding observed by staff causing audible choking/aspiration, in addition to forceful hydration causing audible choking/aspiration;

- Incident of patient's enteral feed bottle not being changed for so long the content had become foul and coagulated; date and expiration of contents not noted on bottle;
- Residents not bathed for several weeks;
- Forceful and aggressive transfers;
- Little/no regular turning of patients leading to increased and more complex pressure ulcers;
- Patients observed crying for help with staff not responding (for 30 min to over 2 hours);
- Regular wellness checks suboptimal or inconsistent, resulting in many hours between checks;
- Incident of permanent catheter being in situ for 3 weeks beyond scheduled change date;
- Significant lack of appropriate wound care leading to advanced (stage 4/unstageable) wounds.

3. Orchard Villa: Pickering, Ontario (for-profit facility)

- Lack of cleanliness noted, cockroaches and flies present; rotten smelly food observed;
- Multiple falls, without required assessment and treatment of pain;
- Inappropriate PPE use noted throughout all staffing levels (doctors included);
- No accountability for staff in regards to upholding basic care needs or best practices;
- Patients being left in beds with soiled incontinence pads rather than being ambulated to toilets;
- Mouth care and hydration schedule not adhered to;

- Staff putting food and important belongings outside of residents' reach;
- Nurses appeared to document assessments without actually having assessed the resident;
- Lack of knowledge regarding what qualifies as restraint: Multiple scenarios of walking aids being removed, or mattresses set on floor as patients were unable to stand from that low position. This was to prevent them from wandering the facility;
- Lack of proper positioning for meals/fluids; staff failing to consistently sit residents up before feeding/ hydrating/giving meds which increased risk of choking/aspiration; including an incident that appeared to have contributed to a resident's death;
- Nursing medication administration errors.

4. Altamont Care Community: Scarborough, Ontario (for-profit facility)

- Medications reported/documented as being given when they were not;
- Inadequate nutrition – due to significant staffing issues, most residents were not given 3 meals per day and there was a significant delay in meals;
- Insufficient wound care;
- Significant number of residents have pressure ulcers, stage 2, 3, and 4 and unstageable as a result of prolonged bed rest;
- Many residents bed bound for several weeks; no evidence of residents being moved to wheelchairs for parts of the day, repositioned in bed, or washed properly;

- A non-verbal resident wrote a disturbing letter alleging neglect and abuse by a PSW. The letter was handed to a CAF member by the resident and then immediately reported to management;
- Scheduling a significant concern; PSW ratio often 1 per wing (30–40+ residents per PSW);
- Current staff-to-patient ratio does not allow for more than the most basic daily requirements.

5. Holland Christian Homes Grace Manor: Brampton, Ontario (not-for-profit facility)

- Staff moving from COVID+ unit to other units without changing contaminated PPE;
- Some staff not following infection prevention and control (IPAC) policies;
- Wearing same pair of gloves for several tasks from one patient to another;
- Standards of practice/quality of care concerns including wound care, medication administration, improper documentation regarding patient DNR status;
- Concerns about agency staff, including:
  - leaving food in a resident's mouth while they were sleeping,
  - aggressively repositioning a resident and improper use of lifts; and
  - not assisting residents during meals (staff would rather write the resident refused to eat, rather than helping them to eat).

These powerful depictions were documented in plain sight and underscored the substandard care provided in far too many LTC homes during the COVID-19 pandemic. It also raises the following questions: What was happening inside LTC homes where the military was not present to observe? How much worse was it without this external supervision? Despite these reports focusing on a handful of Ontario-based LTC homes, they brought the nation to a standstill. Politicians of all stripes held press conferences demanding change, including the prime minister himself. For a moment, there was hope that real change to address the long-standing deficiencies in LTC would occur. It was a rare moment in time when everyone was watching and demands for change could not be easily ignored. I felt immense pressure to strike while the iron was hot, so to speak.

To that end, I provided over 300 news media interviews critiquing provincial and national LTC policies; continued meeting with and sharing accounts from staff and families across Canada on my social media; attended and helped organize protests outside LTC facilities that were battling outbreaks; published editorials in the area; co-created two different advocacy organizations and launched their related advocacy campaigns; testified ahead of the LTC Commission of Ontario pertaining to the impact of pandemic policies on essential family caregivers of loved ones in LTC homes; spoke in front of the Standing Committee at the Legislative Assembly in response to Ontario's Bill 37: Providing More Care, Protecting Seniors, and Building More Beds Act, 2021; participated in a filmed LTC panel for the television show *The Agenda*; ran a series of public town halls

with families, elected officials, front-line staff, and researchers from across Canada as part of an advocacy campaign
for national standards in LTC; and even addressed Prime
Minister Trudeau on this last point while participating in
a pan-Canadian COVID-19 roundtable spearheaded by
Dr. Nili Kaplan-Myrth.[20] All of this was done on a volunteer
basis while working full-time as a professor and conducting
and publishing the results of my own COVID-19–related
research alongside Dr. Charlene Chu that focused on the
trauma that blanket visitation bans were having on essential family caregivers of loved ones in LTC facilities during
the pandemic.[21] To say it was a stressful time would be putting it mildly, but I wouldn't change a thing.

After Everything That Happened, We Must Have Fixed the Problems in LTC, Right?

One would hope that after watching the worst mass casualty
in our collective long-term care history unfold in real time,
we would have come together to fix the known problems in
this sector. Yet little was done to address its systemic flaws.
Not only did Canada repeat the same mistakes as Italy did
at the outset of the pandemic, but also nearly 4 million LTC
residents went on to contract COVID-19 and 40,000 and
counting died as a result.[22] Critical staffing shortages remain. Worse, most provinces are choosing to expand upon
the dysfunctional status quo instead of enacting sweeping
changes so desperately needed, starting with phasing out
private, for-profit LTC.

In Canada, there are 2,076 LTC homes, all of which are publicly funded but their *ownership* is divided into either public or private, with different jurisdictions having different proportions of each. There are LTC homes that are run by governments (i.e., municipal), and there are two kinds of privately owned LTC homes: not-for-profit (e.g., charitable) and for-profit facilities. Overall, 54 per cent of LTC homes in Canada are privately owned and 46 per cent are publicly owned. During COVID-19, researchers found that government-run/public facilities had far fewer deaths than all private (not-for-profit and for-profit) LTC facilities, with for-profit facilities having the worst outcomes.[23] Even before COVID-19, there was significant domestic and international research warning against for-profit LTC, whose corporations have been found to hire less staff, pay their staff less, provide fewer hours of direct care to residents per day, have more transfers to hospitals, more cases of bed ulcers, and use more precariously employed part-time or casual workers, which has led to a serious deterioration in the labour conditions inside these facilities.[24] Ownership matters when it comes to LTC outcomes.

In Ontario, the province with the greatest share of for-profit ownership (58 per cent) compared to private, not-for-profit (24 per cent) and public, municipal (16 per cent),[25] for-profit LTC homes reported 7.3 COVID-19 deaths per 100 registered LTC beds while private, not-for-profit facilities reported 3.8 deaths, and public (municipal) LTC homes reported only 1.5 deaths per 100 beds – a pattern that held even when omitting the ten homes with the highest death rates in the province.[26] What's worse are the findings that while deaths were mounting, which were often linked to critical PPE and staffing shortages in LTC homes, three of the largest for-profit LTC chains paid out nearly $171 million to shareholders at the same time they received $138.5 million in provincial pandemic pay.[27] Evidently, it was more important to divvy out profits to shareholders than to divest those monies to hire staff, purchase life-saving PPE and IPAC support, or provide sick pay so that workers did not feel pressured to go to work sick and risk the lives of residents, a fact that was known by government officials and admitted to by the chief medical health officer at the time, Dr. David Williams.[28]

Even the Ontario commission into LTC homes, launched by the government of Premier Doug Ford in late 2020, reiterated the existence of "numerous studies over the past two decades" that demonstrate poorer resident outcomes and reduced quality of care in for-profit LTC homes compared to not-for-profit LTC homes.[29] Natalie Mehra, director of the Ontario Health Coalition, and I also penned an opinion piece for the *Toronto Star* about how keeping for-profit LTC would be a deadly mistake.[30] It is no wonder that a national movement began that continues today to end for-profit LTC across Canada. There is no doubt in my mind that until we phase out for-profit LTC, any efforts towards improving the sector will be successively undermined by the profit motive. Profit has no place in LTC, and that is the proverbial hill that I will die on.

Despite the glaring evidence against for-profit LTC, Ontario's provincial government has decided to perpetuate the for-profit stronghold in the sector, knowing full well that most COVID-19 deaths occurred in these facilities. Like other provinces, Ontario has begun the process of granting generational licences (i.e., twenty-five to thirty years) to many of the for-profit nursing home chains with the worst COVID-19 death rates.[31] Ontario is choosing to acquiesce instead of taking bold action like Saskatchewan, a province that decided to end its contract with Extendicare (a national private, for-profit LTC chain) and fold those facilities into the public sector after a deadly outbreak occurred in one of its LTC homes.[32] Frankly, this was the time for Canada to learn from everything that happened during the pandemic, heed the long-standing evidence in the area, and ban all future for-profit LTC ownership. It is also what Canadians want, with recent national polling data showing overwhelming support for making all LTC facilities public and not-for-profit.[33] Governments should have jumped to legislate the expansion of only public (government-run) and not-for-profit LTC going forward. Instead, most chose to preserve the existing status quo, sentencing future generations to the same fate.

So What Now?

I wish I could tell everyone that everything has improved and that we are in a better place than we were when the pandemic began. Apart from vaccinations thankfully reducing mass mortality among LTC residents, not much else has changed. Federal and provincial governments continue to fail those who live and work in LTC facilities. The sweeping structural reform that was needed remains outstanding. But as someone once told me when I wanted to give up after seeing so little improvement, you must keep pushing. Progress can be slow and frustratingly incremental before it finally happens, but it can happen. It must happen.

So please, keep using your voices. Every single one of you. At some point, God willing (as my grandfather would always say), you will reach the age where you need LTC; it behoves us all to fix it now.

For families soon to enter the LTC system, I leave you with tips I have learned throughout my advocacy journey that may help you navigate your LTC journey. They are by no means exhaustive, but hopefully, they can help you prepare for what lies ahead:

1 Research your choices for long-term care homes. Who owns the LTC home? For-profit? Not-for-profit? Municipal? What are the public inspection records like for the home? Be aware that many not-for-profit LTC homes also contract out their management to for-profit firms,[34] so enquiring about the home's management is key.

2 Prepare to set up cable and/or a telephone line in your loved one's room. These are not included and remain the responsibility of the resident/their family to install.

3 Make sure you are provided with a clear care plan upon admission and make it known which family members/ friends will be the formal substitute decision-makers and/or contact persons for the resident.

4 Familiarize yourself with the Resident's Bill of Rights
   or any other documents pertaining to the rights of you
   and your loved one in care. Ask the home to provide
   these to you directly, ideally via email or hard copy.
5 Consider putting in a Wi-Fi–enabled camera or tablet
   in your loved one's room to promote added con-
   nectivity and to provide peace of mind in your absence. Family-installed camera footage has also been
   upheld in Canadian courts and has helped secure
   criminal convictions of employees caught abusing
   residents.[35]
6 Visit the home often and get to know as many other
   LTC families and front-line staff as you can. Building
   connections within the LTC is invaluable.
7 Beware that personal items are often lost, even stolen,
   in LTC homes, including wedding rings and other valuable and often irreplaceable items. Copying valuable
   photos and replacing valuable jewellery with cheaper
   duplicates is wise.
8 Join a family council for your LTC home and, if one
   does not exist, consider creating one with help from the
   various Family Council organizations in your province
   (e.g., in Ontario, "Family Councils Ontario" can help).
9 While addressing complaints in-person is good,
   putting them in writing in email form is better. These
   emails should be sent to the director of care and/or facility administrator for your LTC home. Note:
   Written complaints tend to be considered formal
   complaints that must be investigated by LTC
   oversight bodies.

10 If your loved one in LTC requires additional care to
prevent hospitalizations, you can enquire about various funding streams that LTC providers can apply for.
These are rarely advertised by providers, so you will
need to enquire about any additional governmental
funding available to prevent issues like falls, wounds,
and oral care infections. In Ontario, one such fund is re-
ferred to as a "High-Intensity Needs Fund."[36]

11 If your complaints are not dealt with by the home or
keep recurring, lodge formal complaints and request
inspections with whatever reporting outlets are available to you in your province. Be it an LTC action line,
a Patient Ombudsman, or even the police. Depending
on the severity of the issue, keeping a running list of
problems is important for the individual as well as for
demanding institutional change.

12 Routinely ask for a record of the medications provided
to your loved one in the LTC home. Ask for those lists
periodically to make sure there are no unnecessary
interventions being provided without your consent.
There is a known and troubling pattern of "chemical
restraint" in nursing homes, whereby the use of psy-
choactive medications not required for treating medical
symptoms are used to inhibit a person's behaviour or
movement.[37]

13 If the system fails you and your loved one is harmed
due to negligence, civil litigation is an option. Personal injury lawyers can help and, if legal fees are
a concern, there are many who will only take a fee
once they are successful in litigating your case.

Furthermore, successful cases often prompt insurance companies to demand certain improvements from the LTC home as a condition of continued insurance coverage.

I pray that current and future generations of residents have a good LTC experience. I really do hope that you never need to reach out to me or others for help. Unfortunately, the odds are that you will run into issues, so I urge you to be prepared and to know your rights. Stand your ground and please remember not to blame yourselves if anything goes wrong. Too many families confide in me that they are left with overwhelming and often debilitating guilt for "putting them [their loved one] in LTC." I urge you to remember it was never actually a choice given your circumstances and the lack of appropriate infrastructure to help your loved one age at home safely and independently. We would all choose to keep our loved ones in their own homes if it were an option available to us. Every single time.

If I can leave you with some personal advice, it would be to remind you that your voice is powerful. You *can* effect change, and wins were indeed made by speaking up during the COVID-19 pandemic. One big win was the Essential Caregiver Policy that came into effect in September 2020, a policy I believe would not have come into effect without us collectively fighting for it day in and day out. This policy allowed LTC residents in Ontario to designate up to two "essential" caregivers that could visit irrespective of outbreak status, provided they underwent COVID-19 screening and testing, completed infection control training, and abided by safety protocols involving the use of PPE, and so on. This policy was the earliest and most comprehensive of its kind to come into effect across Canada pertaining to the resumption of in-person visitation in LTC homes.[38]

At the end of the day, advocacy is not easy and can be personally and professionally challenging, but it *is* worth it. I am reminded of that whenever someone tells me they became an LTC advocate because of my advocacy. Knowledge is power and the more that gets out there, the better the odds are that change will occur. For far too long, LTC has operated under the public radar, shrouded in secrecy and silence. I wish to break it wide open, but I'll need your help to do it.

DR. VIVIAN STAMATOPOULOS is an Associate Teaching Professor at Ontario Tech University. She holds a Master of Arts (Sociology) and a Doctor of Philosophy (Sociology) from York University. Her research interests focus on child and youth-based caregiving (young carers), unpaid family caregiving, and long-term care (LTC). She is a leading advocate for LTC residents in Ontario, providing over 300 expert interviews on the topic during the COVID-19 pandemic. For her research and advocacy, she has received numerous honours, including The Orville Thacker Award (Ontario Health Coalition, 2022), Ontario Vaccine Hero (*Toronto Star*, 2021), Health Hero (*Best Health* magazine, 2021), Doris Anderson Award (*Chatelaine* magazine, 2021), and the Safety Leadership Award (Ontario Trial Lawyers Association, 2021).

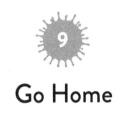

Go Home

KIMIKO SHIBATA

My father used to tell me that I would have to work twice as hard as my classmates to prove myself because I was a girl. Then twice as hard again because I was Asian. He had a huge chip on his shoulder about how he had been treated as a newcomer, both as an international student in the United States and as an immigrant who chose Canada as his forever home. I remember my dad telling me how the KKK threatened him because he dared to work for the Catholic School Board in London, Ontario. How a hotel manager wouldn't rent a room to him because he wasn't white. I remember him wondering aloud if it was his résumé or his accent that prevented him from ever becoming a department head at his school.

As a young teen, I remember thinking that he was stuck in the 1970s. Couldn't he see how much better the world was since he had first come to North America? How much more inclusive Canadian society was? How sexism and racism were not problems we had to worry about anymore? I truly believed what my teachers had told me: that everyone had equal rights and opportunities, and that racism was not a problem in Canada. They were so wrong.

I recognize that my personal experiences of racism during the pandemic have been extremely mild compared to many others. I have not had anyone shoot me for being Asian. I have not had anyone punch or kick me for being Asian. I have not been assaulted for wearing a mask, which is sadly a common occurrence given the relationship between anti-Asian racism and anti-mask sentiment. I have not had people hold me down to cough and spit in my face because they blame me for bringing the virus to Canada. I have not had people vandalize or otherwise damage my property because I am Asian.

I recognize how very lucky I've been throughout this pandemic as someone who holds a steady job and who does not suffer from the intergenerational trauma that haunts the children of Japanese internment camp survivors. I do not have to worry about housing or food insecurity or being the victim of violent hate crimes. I offer you my musings from a place of privilege.

One evening as I was packing my child's lunch for school, I hesitated to put in the toasted nori that she loves. I caught myself thinking that it was pretty much the most "Asian" thing in the world ... eating seaweed. I thought about how this might single her out as belonging to a group that has been actively targeted during this pandemic. And I hate that my mind went there. I hate that I hesitated, even for a moment, to give my child a healthy treat because it may look "too Asian." But I did hesitate. I did pause.

I remembered when a man yelled at my daughter and me to "take the Goddamned virus back with you to China!" as we walked in downtown Kitchener.

> *"Why is that man being so loud, Momma? It's hurting my ears."*
> *"He's really angry. Let's just go home and give him some space."*

I remembered how a man almost hit me with his car as I was walking on the sidewalk, just so that he could roll down the window to yell out "Go back to your own country!"

I remembered being told "Go back to your s-hole country" on social media when someone disagreed with one of my posts.

I remembered, when walking in a store, how someone started to loudly complain to their friend about having to be in the same store as me, as they did not "want to get the China virus from that f-ing Chink." I thought of how I literally froze, unable to speak, then fled the store as quickly as possible, so that I could weep in the safety of my car.

I remembered just about every principal mispronouncing my name whenever I started at a new school, and then having all the other staff follow suit, even if they had originally pronounced it correctly.

I remembered being transferred to a rural school largely populated by Mennonites. The students would gather around me at recess, pointing and laughing because they had never seen someone "who looked like me."

I remembered being asked "Where are you from?" so many times, and people rarely accepting my answers of "southwestern Ontario" or "Canada."

I remembered the question "What country are you from?" when I was out for dinner with a white friend who had immigrated to Canada from the Netherlands. He was amused that nobody ever asked him where he was from, but everyone always seemed to ask me.

I remembered the teacher in school who told the rest of the class that they should just call me "Kim."

I remembered a boy in high school telling me my eyes went "back to my ears" and using his fingers to stretch out the corner of his eyes, and how when I left the room to cry in the hallway, I was sent to the office for disrupting the class and was suspended for the rest of the day as punishment.

I remembered elementary school classmates asking me if I spoke "Ching Chong" and making "Ching Chong" noises at me on the schoolyard while teachers gave their students a lesson in being bystanders.

I remembered children chanting "Dirty knees, Japanese" in a skipping rhyme.

I remembered the other kids at daycare asking why my skin was darker than theirs and feeling ashamed. "Tell them you have a suntan," my mom said.

These tiny experiences form a thick uninterrupted line of anti-Asian racism. These moments and memories still live in our bodies and in our brains, and they are triggered when we are scared to send our children to school with nori. In twenty-first-century Canada!

I am stunned at the number of anti-Asian experiences that I see in the media. Social media has given racists an open platform.

On 16 March 2021, I was pummelled by the stories about Asian women being murdered in Atlanta. I cried myself to sleep. How could I feel safe in my Asian body?

In May 2021, a family not too far from my home woke up to rocks being thrown through their windows with messages on them: "You bring COVID, move out." I didn't leave the house without my husband for several days. When I did leave the house, I wore sunglasses to cover my Asian eyes.

According to Statistics Canada, the number of police-reported Asian hate crimes increased by 301 per cent in 2020.[1] When former US president Donald Trump started calling COVID-19 the "China Virus" and the "Chinese Virus" in March of 2020 on television and on social media, he unleashed a wave of hatred towards people of Asian descent, starting with anti-Asian hashtags on Twitter that encouraged people to engage in hate crimes and overt anti-Asian racism. Although the World Health Organization tried to convince people not to tie the virus to a specific ethnicity or geographical location, the damage had already been done. People had found their scapegoat for the pandemic, and they were emboldened and united in their hatred.

Being a person of Asian descent during this pandemic has added a whole new layer of stress onto an already challenging time. Overt anti-Asian racism has been rearing its ugly head globally and within my own community, and any shred that I may have had left of my childhood wishful thinking that racism was not a problem in Canada anymore has been destroyed.

The pandemic didn't cause anti-Asian racism. It just made the existing racism more visible and, frankly, more socially acceptable. The good news is that when something is made visible, it can be recognized and treated. Now is the time to treat the virus of racism.

As an educator, I am in a unique position in which I can help children to unlearn their own biases and misunderstandings about race. Just before lockdown in 2020, I heard my students say:

"My mom says we can't go to a hotel trip for March Break because China people will make us sick and they closed down all the airports."

"My dad says Chinese eat bats and that's why people are dying. Do you eat bats, Ms. Shibata? I don't want you to die."

"If you eat Chinese food, you will get coronavirus."

We changed our lesson that day to learn about how viruses actually spread and how to protect ourselves from getting sick or spreading illness. We spoke about how viruses do not belong to a country, culture, or ethnicity, nor are they the fault of any particular group of people.

Thankfully, my students felt safe enough in my classroom to voice their concerns, so that I could help them understand the facts. Kids pick up on the fear and prejudice of the adults around them. We need to encourage them to ask questions even when their words are uncomfortable. The goal should never be to shut down the conversation, but rather to actively promote truth over fear. Accurate information and courageous conversations with children are our first line of defence against racism in our schools and communities.

To my allies who want to know how they can help:

- Anti-racism work is both urgent and necessary. Awareness of racism is important, but don't stop there.
- Actively work to dismantle racism in your systems, your workplaces, your schools, and your communities.
- Question policies that advantage the dominant group.
- Question "the way things have always been done."
- Ask people what they need and what barriers they are facing, and then focus on listening to hear instead of listening to respond.
- Be willing to feel uncomfortable.
- Have courageous conversations.
- Be humble.
- Be willing to make mistakes and apologize.
- Be willing to de-centre yourself in the work.

And remember that if my child is old enough to have racist slurs thrown at her, then your child is old enough to learn that racism exists. Active as opposed to performative allyship is needed now, more than ever. The time for talking about racism is over. What can you do to disrupt and change the very systems that benefit you?

To my fellow racialized friends who are hurting right now: Do not be small. Do not be invisible. Tell your stories. Celebrate your cultures and your languages. Do not lose yourselves. In the past, I have chosen safety over confrontation when it comes to racism. No longer.

I refuse to be invisible. I refuse to lock down my Twitter account to avoid more attacks. I will hold my head high and be fully present and visible in my community. I will celebrate my cultural identity. I will correct the pronunciation of my name, especially when the person mispronouncing it is the leader in the room. I don't want my child to grow up in fear. I don't want her to ever feel like she has to hide a part of herself. I want her to be proud of who she is. I will pack my daughter that nori she loves and throw in some sushi for good measure.

KIMIKO SHIBATA has been an educator in both childcare and elementary school classroom settings. She is currently an MLL (Multilingual Language Learner) resource teacher for the Waterloo Region District School Board in Ontario, and enjoys helping colleagues use technology to make learning and communication more equitable and accessible for multilingual students and their caregivers.

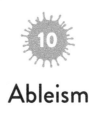

Ableism

KENZIE McCURDY

Spring 2022.

Remember back in 2020, during that first COVID-19 lockdown, how everyone was talking about pollution declining and how the ozone layer was healing? Interspersed with the anxiety and fear of getting sick, we watched infection numbers rise around the world, but there were hopeful conversations about how maybe we could learn something from this virus. Maybe it would make the world a better place, and make us better people.

Disabled people knew that wasn't going to happen. And it didn't.

Prime Minister Justin Trudeau spoke to Canada daily. He told us he'd have our backs, and that no one would be left behind. As they watched him talk through the screen each day, disabled Canadians grew more and more on edge. Help for employers, help for employees, help for students, help for seniors. They watched anxiously, waiting for their turn.

It didn't come.

During those first months of the pandemic, I was off work, at home, and using social media more than usual. I started to notice people talking about their pandemic experiences. The disabled Twitter community was outraged:

> *"They've forgotten us!"*
> *"No, they've not forgotten us, they're ignoring us."*
> *"They want us dead!"*
> *"They won't give us money, but they'll give us medical assistance in dying (MAID)!"*

I started to retweet these comments and engage others in dialogue about disability poverty. The more I saw, the more disturbed I became. I wasn't prepared for how difficult it would be to make this topic heard.

> *"Those people were already on disability assistance. Their situation didn't change, so why should they get more money?"*

I began to pay more attention to Twitter and to what disabled users were saying. They were having a much rougher time surviving during the pandemic than they were before. And let me tell you, they were hardly getting by pre-pandemic! Not only were those receiving social assistance continuing to live 40 per cent below the poverty line,[1] they now had added costs they didn't have to worry about before: gloves, masks, and hand sanitizer. Many had to have their groceries delivered and take taxis instead of public transit because they were immunocompromised. Leaving their home had become a risk many didn't want to take.

Some fellow disabled Twitter users and I got together to try to bring some attention to the situation. One of the first things we did was to approach the media. We were completely stunned by the reaction we received. Nobody thought disability poverty was newsworthy. We were told by the media: "We don't make the news, we just report it. We don't see people rising up and complaining. There are no marches in the street."

The most vulnerable population – those with medical issues or who are immunosuppressed; those who are poor; those who rely on para transit, caregivers, or attendant care – they're supposed to go out and march, in the middle of a pandemic, to let people know how poorly they're doing? This was our first brush with ableism in the media and we called them out. They responded by saying that they didn't think it was ableism. We went back and forth a couple of times but eventually they just stopped responding to us. If only they could see, would look at, what we experience in real life every single day.

We eventually did get some media to see the issue and report on it, but the stories were not framed the way we wanted. Nobody owned the fact that the Government of Canada and provincial governments were practising full-blown ableism. In their eyes, disabled Canadians on social assistance were already being helped so they could push them aside while they attended to all the working people.

Then the Canada Emergency Response Benefit (CERB) happened. A quick $2,000 a month to anyone whose job was lost because of COVID-19. No questions asked. Months later when it became known that many people had applied and received CERB erroneously, the federal government said it would not make any effort to recover the lost money. The government was moving on. With that statement, the government had just told disabled people three things: they were willing to waste money on working Canadians; that the basic monthly income they saw people needing, in this economy, was $2,000; and that they felt it was reasonable to keep disabled individuals who were not able to work, through no fault of their own, 40 per cent below that number.[2]

Eventually, news outlets started reporting sporadically some stories about disabled poverty. Trudeau even went so far as to introduce a Canadian Disability Benefit. He dangled it like a carrot by way of the Throne Speech, then swiftly pulled it up and away, out of reach when he decided to call an election. It took over a year to get it reintroduced. And even a year and a half later, it was an empty outline going through Parliament to see if people really did need such a benefit. There was no such process for CERB.

So here we are, over two years into a worldwide pandemic and people on the Ontario Disability Support Program are not only applying to MAID, but they are getting accepted. Their dire poverty is making their lives so miserable, so unbearable, that they just want out. And the MAID criteria keep widening. We have a federal government that legislates poverty for the disabled and then makes it easy and legal for you to end your own life because of that poverty. Canada, the land of the free. Except if you're disabled; then there's a very, very high cost.

The federal government must do more, and quickly, to protect Canada's disabled population. Disabled Canadians need more money directly in their hands so that they are in control of their own health and safety. The federal government needs to recognize that by keeping disabled Canadians close to 40 per cent below the poverty line, it is saying that it's not willing to invest in human beings who, through no fault of their own, cannot work. But not only does the government need to get the money out as quickly as possible, it needs to do it with some certainty that the provinces will not claw the benefits back as a result. And, if it's meant to lift people out of poverty, it really needs to do just that, not bring them from severe, devastating, soul-crushing, health-destroying poverty to poverty, but actually out of poverty. Full stop.

How many people need to die before the government does something? How many studies need to be done before it's convinced that poverty and ableism are killing our disabled community?

And most importantly, who will hold the government accountable for those who have already died?

KENZIE McCURDY grew up in Montreal and now works as a social worker at the Ottawa Hospital. She is passionate about equality and accessibility. She is co-coordinator for the Ottawa chapter of the StopGap Foundation, which builds accessibility ramps for businesses with single-step entrances. Kenzie is also part of a women's poetry group.

Still Here

REVEREND CANON MAGGIE HELWIG

April 2022.

We're still here, I say, when people ask how I am. *We're still doing what we do.*

For years, my little downtown church in Toronto has been running a drop-in, dinner, and breakfasts for people who are homeless, inadequately housed, hungry, or just lonely.

On one weekend in March 2020, every support in the city on which our guests had depended vanished overnight: Out of the Cold programs, most drop-ins, libraries, late-night Tim Hortons or McDonald's, everything except the Toronto Transit Commission, whose buses, streetcars, and subways became a sort of travelling emergency shelter as most other people stopped using them. My church, along with a handful of other drop-ins around the city, remained open. We served pizza slices rescued from events that had been suddenly cancelled. That Friday night, people sat in the church crying because it was the first time they'd been able to sit down for days. One man tore our back door off the hinges half an hour before we opened. Outside, two people fought in the road, police cars everywhere, everyone desperate, terrified, angry.

We had one box of surgical masks, and no idea when or how we might get our hands on another. A volunteer started baking twenty loaves of bread a week, because the supermarkets had been cleared out, and when bread arrived on the shelves, there were quotas, and we had no way to prove that we were preparing hundreds of meals. The bishop sent us letters to carry with us, verifying that we were required to work outside our homes, and required to travel to and from work, in case we were stopped, though of course that was never a real threat. But for a while, there seemed to be no knowing what might happen.

Two years later, we have N95s and rapid tests from the City of Toronto, though the supply is unpredictable and confusing, and some of my colleagues at other drop-ins still have nothing. My volunteers have been through the Alpha wave and the Delta wave and the Omicron wave, and some of them have family members with long COVID, and some of our guests are now in housing, and some are dead, but most are still here, still struggling. We run vaccine clinics and information sessions, swimming against a rip tide of disinformation. I have led church services on Zoom while a red-tailed hawk roosted on the fence outside my window. I have held funerals out of doors in the wind, or with all the church windows open in late December. *We're still here.*

I begin one spring day trying to help the police identify a dead man in a doorway at Dundas and Kensington. Another day, someone is lying dead in the park. Overdose, the other pandemic. Sometimes when I'm cycling to work in the morning, I see city crews in the park, ripping up tents with knives.

I always supposed that I might grow up to live in a dystopian future, but I was younger then, and thought it would be more exciting than it is.

Two years in, I watch my life shrinking as the world decides to open wide up, as capacity limits and mask mandates disappear. The empty storefronts in the neighbourhood are covered with anti-mask/anti-vaxx graffiti, and "freedom" protests still march to Queen's Park every Saturday, with their sea of Canadian flags and their bizarre conspiracy placards, though they now have everything they claim to have wanted.

My priorities have always been to avoid making my vulnerable guests sick, and to protect, as far as I can, my disabled adult daughter, but the choices I must make now are different. I do not attend my own installation as an honorary canon of the St. James Cathedral. I do not attend a city hall event recognizing the work of the Vaccine Engagement Teams, even though I am prouder of this work than of almost anything else I have ever done. I do not travel to see my increasingly frail mother in Kingston. My husband sets his alarm so he can get into stores as soon as they open to buy our groceries.

Will the City of Toronto continue to supply us with masks after the mandate for drop-ins ends? We have no idea.

We research how many times you can safely reuse an N95. Across the street, there's a coffee shop full of unmasked people, enjoying what they believe, in all good faith, to be the "post-pandemic era."

It really shouldn't bother me that people who didn't leave their houses during the first wave now accuse me of being fearful because I wear a mask indoors, but it does bother me sometimes, and I mutter in my head about how I have travelled in war zones and broken up bar fights between men twice my size, as if this made me a better person somehow.

I sit on the grimy floor of the parish hall with a man in alcohol withdrawal, waiting for the paramedics, and I think that this quiet time in a dimly lit room is one of the least stressful moments I've had for weeks.

It is all fragments; there is no conclusion to this. I can't write a proper ending to this piece because nothing is ending.

We are still here.

MAGGIE HELWIG (she/they) is a settler in the territory of the Dish With One Spoon wampum belt covenant. She is the author of a number of books of poetry and fiction; her novel *Girls Fall Down* (Coach House Press, 2008) was shortlisted for the City of Toronto Book Award. She is also an Anglican priest at the Church of St. Stephen-in-the-Fields in Kensington Market, which provides extensive programming for homeless, underhoused, and food-insecure community members.

The Pandemic Changed Nothing (for Worse and Better)

MEAGAN GILLMORE

Mere weeks after the World Health Organization declared the novel coronavirus a worldwide emergency, transfixing the world around me with stories of disaster, I felt restless and detached. Lockdowns plunged my days into repetitive predictability, and I found it difficult to know what stories deserved my attention.

It was embarrassing to admit this out loud. As a journalist, I was, technically, an essential worker, and there was no shortage of stories in the spring of 2020. Each daily press conference with Prime Minister Justin Trudeau was a cornucopia of questions to ask and responses to dissect: How was the government making decisions? Would the rationale be explained? Who would be the first to make a "speaking moistly" meme? And then there was the question I repeated most often to myself: What support would there be for disabled Canadians?

The overwhelming silence revealed the reason why I found the whole catastrophe so monotonous: for disabled Canadians, like myself and many of the people I encounter in my work, nothing had changed.

The indifference to disability hurt. By no means was it unprecedented, to borrow the buzzword of 2020. But, for a moment, I'd thought the pandemic would break the long-established precedent of disabled citizens being overlooked in emergency responses. During the months preceding the pandemic, there were signs that Canada was moving into a new era in disability rights. The year 2020 had dawned with plenty of optimism – and puns about seeing clearly. In some ways, for disabled Canadians who follow public policy about disability, the positivity was clearly warranted. Canada's first federal accessibility legislation, the Accessible Canada Act, had come into force in July 2019 and had garnered unanimous support in the House of Commons. Accessibility Standards Canada, the organization tasked with creating standards under the new law, was primed to begin its work in earnest. Even changing federal minister Carla Qualtrough's title from Minister of Accessibility to Minister of Disability Inclusion[1] signalled an emphasis on having disabled Canadians enjoy full equality throughout society. There was a sense that perhaps this government would make real and tangible progress.

As I plotted out my workplans for the year, reporting on disability policy for Accessible Media Inc., a national not-for-profit broadcaster dedicated to reporting about disability stories and policy, I envisioned explaining the development of new policies that could greatly benefit people's lives. I wondered if disability coverage would receive greater prominence. (Admittedly, an egotistical part of me wondered if I would be part of that coverage.)

The pandemic destroyed all that optimism. I spent the first few months providing weekly updates about the difficulties disabled Canadians were having accessing services and their concerns with the solutions that were being proposed. I talked to individuals who wondered how their physical needs would be met when everyone was being told to stay away; parents who were struggling to access programs, supports, and education for their children; disability organizations that were trying to keep all their members connected. Over and over, I asked, "What's changed for you?"

And the answer was always, "Nothing."

And then, my interviewees would elaborate:

- Supports for adults labelled with developmental and intellectual disabilities have always been lacking, and the support systems are cumbersome.
- Disabled students have always struggled to navigate inaccessible education environments.
- Employment is often precarious for workers with disabilities.
- Fears about ableist medical ideologies have always been present.
- And isolation? That's been the constant acquaintance of many disabled Canadians.

Perhaps, I wondered dryly, we were better suited for this pandemic than anyone else.

One could argue that I had been preparing for the job of reporting on disability responses (or non-responses) to public health emergencies for nearly twenty years. A few months before I graduated high school, my mother took me out of an afternoon class for an appointment. We headed to a dingy building in downtown Brantford, Ontario, where an experienced government employee explained to me that when I turned eighteen, I would be eligible to become a recipient of the Ontario Disability Support Program. I only had to complete a pile of forms to be transferred from the supports my parents had been receiving on my behalf to the adult program.

I felt flabbergasted, confused. Betrayed. As far as I knew, everyone in my life who mattered viewed my lifelong visual impairment, at best, as a minor inconvenience that alternatively made it easier for me to get lost and easier to tell jokes, like about the time I doused french fries in soy sauce at a restaurant, mistaking the condiment for malt vinegar. Words like "legally blind" or "severe disability" were just phrases reserved for medical forms; outside of annual visits to the ophthalmologist, it wasn't as if they impacted my everyday life.

The only bright spot in that appointment was the different colours on the forms I had to complete. As my mother and I left, I looked around the waiting room at the people sitting in the stiff chairs. The disability office shared a waiting room with other social assistance programs. I glanced at my mother, wide-eyed, trying to process what I had just learned about my life and where I was. "Mom," I asked, "do some of these people come here every day?"

She nodded. And I vowed to never return to that room, or publicly admit I used the programs administered there.

Throughout the weeks of lockdowns, my mind often travelled back to that mostly forgotten day. Except now, with every article I wrote or broadcast segment I produced, I wanted everyone to see what I had seen that day, to feel the despair I had felt when I'd looked at my future through the lens of meagre social assistance cheques.

Anyone who has ever applied for a government disability support program or service has experienced first-hand the frustration that results when underfunding and an overabundance of bureaucracy collides with the varied impacts of disabilities. The pandemic just revealed that to the rest of the country. While the federal government offered some relief to sectors ranging from aviation to telecommunications to fisheries, and policies were being unveiled for business owners, employees, and tenants, disabled Canadians were wondering when their moment would come. The wait continued. On the Easter 2020 long weekend, the federal government announced the creation of an advisory group to provide Minister Qualtrough with information about disabled Canadians' experiences of the pandemic. The first targeted relief for disabled Canadians – not including policies related to students – wasn't unveiled until June: a one-time payment of $600 for disabled Canadians who received the Disability Tax Credit. It was met with resounding cries of too little, too late and questions about what support there would be for disabled Canadians who were deemed ineligible for the Disability Tax Credit. Ultimately, legislation to create the benefit – which eventually included expanded eligibility[2] – wasn't passed until July 2020. But some individuals didn't receive their payments until that fall.

In the interim, disabled Canadians watched millions of their fellow citizens receive $2,000 a month in Canada Emergency Relief Benefit (CERB) payments. Many lauded the program as an efficient and prompt response to the very real economic needs created by the pandemic and the subsequent lockdowns, but for disabled Canadians, it was a clear, public reminder of the legislated poverty many have lived in for decades. All provincial and territorial disability social assistance programs are much less than $2,000 – in some jurisdictions, regular monthly disability social assistance rates are less than half of the amount CERB offered.[3] And if disability social assistance recipients did qualify for CERB, more often than not, their regular benefits were clawed back as a result. Not only were disabled Canadians often the last to be considered when receiving relief, they were also often further penalized for accessing the exact same benefits non-disabled Canadians were given freely, seemingly with no conditions.

Financial policies provided an easily digestible way to show the disparity that rules the lives of many disabled Canadians – a segment of the population that is significantly more likely to spend the typical working years of 18 to 64 living in poverty – pandemic or not. Statistics Canada data indicate that 28 per cent of 25- to 64-year-olds with more severe disabilities live in poverty, in contrast to the 14 per cent of individuals in the same age range who have milder disabilities. Only 10 per cent of their non-disabled peers live in poverty.[4] But many other pandemic-related policies and responses also disproportionately impacted disabled Canadians in negative ways – and those weren't as well publicized. Parents whose children required intensive at-home medical care were scrambling to find and buy sufficient personal protective equipment for those they had trusted to care for their children. Home-care staffing shortages and worries about transmitting the coronavirus left many parents without outside help, forcing them to become twenty-four-hour nurses – often unpaid labour. And while parents who needed to take time off work to care for family members who were sick with COVID-19 received some benefits, those who had left the workforce years earlier to care for their children with disabilities didn't receive similar support. Visitor restrictions meant disabled individuals who were living in group homes or long-term care facilities were unable to see family or friends, the very people who could help them maintain their mental well-being, and often, ensure they got proper medical care, if needed.

Citizens hope that, during a public health emergency, public health officials will provide clear, accurate information that inspires confidence and comfort. Yet for disabled Canadians, healthcare policies often gave only one clear message: we don't value you enough to care for you. Draft provincial triage protocols indicated that, in some jurisdictions, if there were too few ventilators to meet the demand for them, disabled patients – particularly those labelled as having intellectual or developmental disabilities – would not receive them. The policies, understandably, prompted public outcry and calls for change, but it's not clear how much those calls have been heeded. At the end of August

2022, the Ontario government changed a law governing long-term care so that alternative level of care hospital patients – often seniors or disabled people – could be moved to a long-term care home without having to give their consent.

It's been more than three years since the pandemic began. While many of us have returned to some sort of pre-pandemic life, many disabled Canadians I speak to still acutely feel the worry of the pandemic: not only of contracting a potentially life-threatening disease but also of having their needs overlooked and ignored. And underlying many of these concerns is that fact that, for many, the hardest part of the COVID-19 pandemic has been that it hasn't been the hardest battle disabled Canadians have had to fight. In February 2020, the federal government first introduced significant changes to the sections of the Criminal Code that govern medical assistance in dying (MAID) – often known worldwide as euthanasia or physician assisted suicide. Canadian law has always said that only individuals who have a "serious and incurable illness, disease or disability" and are in an "advanced state of decline in capability" that is causing enduring and intolerable physical or psychological suffering that can't be fixed by any method they deem acceptable can receive MAID. Since its adoption in 2016, critics have warned this unfairly targets disabled Canadians. But they hoped the safeguard that restricted MAID eligibility only to those whose natural deaths were considered "reasonably foreseeable" would keep people safe from untimely deaths due to covert or overt coercion. In February 2020, the government introduced an amendment that would allow MAID to be administered to people whose natural deaths aren't reasonably foreseeable – putting Canadians with chronic illnesses and disabilities at specific risk.[5]

The changes were passed into law in March 2021, shortly after the first anniversary of the COVID-19 pandemic. In that year, many disabled Canadians struggled to secure consistent and appropriate healthcare, many lived in financial insecurity exacerbated by pandemic-related job losses and the often detrimental way federal and provincial benefits interact with each other. Many experienced increased isolation that led to significant decreases in mental health. And still, they fought for each other's lives, and they advocated for their dignity in front of a government that was intent on making it easier for them to die. According to Health Canada, 219 individuals whose natural deaths were not reasonably foreseeable died in 2021; 45 per cent of these individuals had a neurological condition, like multiple sclerosis, ALS, or Parkinson's disease.[6] This happened during the emergencies caused by a global pandemic. Disabled Canadians were again largely left behind during COVID-19 responses. But should that be a surprise when the government was considering legislation that significantly put their lives at risk, even without a pandemic?

If we place the COVID-19 pandemic within a larger context of the fight for disability rights, the lack of government response to disabled Canadians' needs isn't surprising at all. A worldwide pandemic is less destructive than the belief that some people's lives are worth less than others' just because they live with a disability or an illness.

But surely, people want to know, what were the good things that happened? There must be some policies worth replicating. Perhaps. There seems to be progress on a national disability benefit, a financial supplement for eligible disabled Canadians, but it's unclear when people will receive the benefit, or how much the benefit is. The first payments may come partway through 2024, but no one's sure yet. But I don't think change primarily occurs in the halls of government power, or at least, I don't think it begins there. The more I've listened to people's stories about disability policy across this country, the more I've been reminded that meaningful change has only come after many long battles for it, whether that's parents filing human rights complaints so they could, during pandemic restrictions, visit their children who were residing in group homes in a way that's best for them. Years of lobbying has, in some provinces, resulted in laws that support the decision-making capabilities of those with intellectual or developmental disabilities.

That doesn't solve everything. Despite my attempts to deny it at first, my adult life has been marked by government-regulated poverty and restrictions on my income that have produced waves of social shame and isolation.

Yet the pandemic has shown me, in new ways, the vibrancy of the people who often find themselves struggling against restrictive government systems. While reporting about disability policy for various news outlets, I met advocates who are fighting tirelessly to be allowed to live in homes of their choosing. I spoke to parents who describe their disabled children as the strongest people they know – even as their love for their children motivates them to face human rights tribunals, start innovative not-for-profits, and share their vulnerabilities publicly. I met friends who spent countless hours helping their disabled friends who were living in group homes communicate with the wider society. I met disabled Canadians who were caring for each other through social media and in-person social connections. And when a protest descended on my current city, Ottawa, it was my disabled peers who reached out to me to make sure I had everything I needed.

Yes, disabled people have always faced barriers throughout society. The pandemic didn't change that. But we've also found simple and creative ways around them, even as we argue for their destruction.

In that way, the pandemic has allowed us to display a resiliency that flourishes to this day.

MEAGAN GILLMORE is an Ottawa-based journalist with the news site *Canadian Affairs*. She's worked throughout Canada and has reported on disability issues for media outlets, including the *Toronto Star*, *TVO.org*, *Broadview Magazine*, *Chatelaine*, *The Walrus*, and *Accessible Media Inc.* She was nominated for a National Magazine Award in 2022 for a *Broadview Magazine* article about disabled young adults who live in long-term care.

Wild Teens: Youth Mental Health and the Pandemic

DR. GAIL BECK

Just before the beginning of the pandemic in Canada, Canadian teens were starting the second semester of high school. Some were applying to college or university. They were getting ready for March Break. These were my patients. When they came in to see me, they would tell me about the courses they would take. They were trying to decide whether they would live on campus.

There won't be statistics in this chapter to inform you about the extent to which the COVID-19 pandemic affected youth mental health. I am not going to speak about the most serious psychiatric problems we are seeing two years on from when the pandemic started. I won't mention that we don't have the resources to care for the youth affected or even to properly evaluate them. It is much more important for you to be able to understand what children and teens endured emotionally through the pandemic. With this understanding, you will be able to support the youth you know as they recover their mental health.

I am going to ask you to remember what it was like to be a teen yourself. I want you to feel once again the wildness of your own adolescence. Most parents remember their own risk-taking exploits ruefully, often realizing that their own teen is no different from them. The untamed nature of youth was commented on in ancient times by Aristotle when he noted that "all their mistakes are in the direction of doing things excessively and vehemently."[1] Once psychology and sociology progressed, practitioners noted the experimentation and risk-taking of youth. Erik Erikson, in his landmark book on adolescent psychological development, *Identity, Youth, and Crisis*, noted that adolescents often explored customs outside their own upbringing and culture as a means to determine their personal identity.[2] This exploration has always been a matter of concern to parents. As a girl growing up when not many women became doctors, I recall my grandmother and other older relatives worrying about the risk I was taking to commit to many years of education.

Apart from these historical, psychological, and sociological observations, more recent research in neurosciences and brain development has shown structural and physiological differences between teens whose brains are still developing and adults. Studies in functional magnetic resonance imaging (fMRI)[3] have demonstrated variability between adults' and adolescents' brains when making decisions. Parts of adults' brains around the frontal lobes will show increased activity when decisions are being made. The activated part of the brain, the anterior cingulate cortex, is involved in detecting mistakes. This area of the brain is not fully developed in teens and continues to develop into a person's mid-twenties. Risk-taking and thinking through how to act helps a teen learn better ways of doing.

The risks teens take are good for their development and they usually take these risks with their friends. They also usually work out with friends when plans are too poorly thought out. Considering this, we must ask: What was the impact of the isolation that kept teens from each other? I was struck by how many of the teens in my practice noted, "I never thought I'd be so happy to get back to school!"

If we had been serious about protecting teens' mental health during the pandemic, then we would have found ways for them to be young. We would have acknowledged the need to find ways for them to be together and do the ridiculous, foolhardy things that are typical and that help them develop emotionally and intellectually. Why didn't we remember some of the things we did ourselves and figure out how teens could manage these from a safe social distance? Thinking of the various ways in which the pandemic has affected youth, in hindsight there was no greater loss for them than that of safe places in our communities where they could gather and socialize and be their lovely, unfettered selves.

Wise societies have always found ways to allow teens to learn about and develop independence by themselves, but in the relative safety of our communities. Skateboard parks, boys' and girls' clubs, and even the traditional "rumspringa" in Amish communities are all institutions that can provide youth safe spaces to do all the things that are normal for adolescents. With the pandemic limiting getting together outside of "bubbles," teens were denied these opportunities, and this was the greatest source of distress for them. Even worse, we did not have the wisdom as a society to realize this.

Every parent with an adolescent, or who has raised an adolescent, is aware that experimentation, risk-taking, and pushing boundaries are all part of the normal experiences of adolescence. We know this – sometimes to our horror – but we have also always prepared for this by planning community spaces and dances and socials. Even recess and lunch breaks at school, as much as some teens say they dread them, can be delightful opportunities to mingle and talk and solve problems when you have a few friends to spend them with. In the pandemic, the social aspects of recess and lunch breaks disappeared, giving way to eating at your desk to avoid contaminating each other. It was safe, but lonely.

If we had been wiser, we would have realized how isolated teens would be. We might have worked with teens to help them figure out how they could be together to work out all the problems the pandemic posed. Could you have a socially distanced dance somehow? Would the principal help you plan it as a school activity to raise money for charity? How do they plan those drive-by events? Can we have one? Necessity is the mother of invention!

It is possible that, if we had spent more time working out how to bring teens together, adults would have listened to more wild and foolish ideas than usual. As someone who has heard wild ideas from five youth in my home and hundreds of others over years of practice, I thought of this. Parents and teachers thought of it, but in the first months of the pandemic, no one listened. There were too many other stresses to consider: How deadly was the virus? What protection did we need? Would I keep my job? How did I make sure my child wouldn't lose a year of school? Governments shut down schools, effectively shutting down children of all ages and all their needs.

I work in two clinical programs: an inpatient unit for youth and a mental health program in a school. My patients and I see a lot of each other. As well as their individual appointments with me, I join them for meals, play board games, and watch television. As the pandemic progressed, I watched my patients' exuberance disappear. This was especially evident with the youth who were in the online school program, seeing their friends only on a screen. They were so desperate to see each other, they even tried to play board games online.

In the early months of 2020, some of my patients wanted to work in nursing or as paramedics or doctors and they spoke to me about hundreds, thousands, of people dying in China. It was sad to them, but it seemed far removed.

Teens are empathetic and many spoke to me of how difficult it must be to be locked down in your home, with so many people dying. In one breath, they lamented the woes of youth in China, but the next moment I was shown pictures of grad dresses and the college campuses people had visited.

Then COVID-19 spread to Europe. Europe was closer.
Youth were more frightened:

*"Dr. Beck, did you see the news reports of people dying in Italy?
My nona and nono are from Italy and they know people who are
sick with this COVID."*

*"There isn't enough space in hospitals in Italy for all the people
who are sick. Did you hear that, Dr. Beck?"*

The pandemic began for my patients in March 2020.

Not only had families cancelled holidays but no one
could get together with their friends. One patient's grandmother died in a retirement residence.

School was cancelled and my patients wondered,
"Am I going to graduate? Am I going to be able to go to
university?"

No one had an answer. "Don't worry. We'll refund your
money." That's what they were told.

But they heard, "Don't worry. We'll refund your life."
Because everyone knew that their lives could be ruined
forever.

When the pandemic precautions first began in March
2020 in Canada, many families were strong and the people
in those families thrived initially. Most of these families
had a reasonable source of income. Parents began to work
from home and the stress of everyone getting up, getting
ready, getting out the door, getting home, getting supper,
and getting to bed all disappeared. Those families suddenly had some big burdens dropped from their day.

But other families were in trouble. These were the families with marginal incomes or serious problems, problems like abuse or chronic illness or poverty. In families with these problems, it did not take long for the abuse to get worse, for the illnesses to become serious, and for the poverty to mean that children had no way to join the virtual school. Even when the teachers could drop off a Chromebook – and many teachers I know did drop off Chromebooks – there were families who could not afford the cost of internet for kids to attend school. The problems in these families got worse exponentially during the pandemic and most of the kids from these families have never recovered. There is no therapy that fixes poverty.

Of those youth not affected by poverty or family difficulties, two groups of mental health patients emerged. There were those whose mental health deteriorated immediately and there were those who did well initially and whose mental health got worse later in the pandemic.

I had thought that being out of school would be extremely difficult for all kids, so I was surprised when a group of youth emerged who got better in the first months of the pandemic. These were teens who found the pre-pandemic world difficult. They were the socially anxious, the bullied, the outcasts. Freed from the terror of having to be out in the world, they were able to focus on studying and on hobbies in a way they never had before. When the pandemic began, these youth were stronger, but that didn't last when they had to return to school.

Some of the worst worries youth had were about getting COVID-19. For others, thinking about their peers dying was a wake-up call:

"Dr. Beck, did you see the story in the news about the nineteen-year-old guy who had COVID-19 and almost died?"

"I did. Wasn't that upsetting?"

"Yes, but I think it will help me not to think about suicide again – at least for a while."

"I'm glad to hear that but tell me how that happened. It might help someone else."

"It's easy to figure out. I was watching TV, listening to this guy talk about how scared he was that he might die and I realized that I owed it to him to stay alive and be glad that I haven't been sick like he was. I don't know this guy or anything, but to me, it's like he's been in hospital frightened of dying and in pain on a respirator. You could tell just listening to him that he was terrified and lonely when he was sick. If he can live with all that, then I will live with my anxiety and depression which is my life-threatening illness, and work to get better. I'm going to do it. Just like he had to fight, I must fight."

I could not think of anything to say. It wasn't necessary. That boy has been well ever since this epiphany and is in college working to become a paramedic.

Not all my patients fared as well. We made the difficult decision to close the inpatient unit. Speaking with youth and their families, we considered that hospitals might not be as safe as home and decided that we would discharge everyone to the safety of home. Daily virtual follow-up was established after a day or two of fumbling with Zoom Healthcare and doxy.me technology that was then unfamiliar. Some who were discharged home continue to struggle even now.

Another group of young psychiatry patients affected were those in day programs. The day hospital program in Youth Psychiatry at my hospital closed its group rooms, activity room, and classrooms in favour of a virtual setting. As schools closed, the various special education programs in schools, including the mental health program, closed. At the same time, all psychiatric outpatient assessments and treatment of children and teens switched to virtual modalities of care. For youth who needed intensive treatment, this was difficult.

When schools reopened and in-person programs returned, many youth were relieved. Relief was short-lived as schools opened and closed and opened and closed. There was a lot of anger at the indecision.

"What is the matter with grown-ups?"
"They didn't listen in science, did they, Dr. Beck?"

We all noticed the inconsistency of the advice provided by governments as to what precautions were necessary and safe. Schools closed, then opened … and then they closed again. Wear masks, don't wear masks – the recommendations changed so often it was impossible to know what to do. For some teens, it was infuriating and tempers flared. For others, discouragement became entrenched. Teens wanted to know what to do and parents were desperate to know how to ensure their kids followed the recommendations.

My experience is that the best interventions, whether you are a parent or a psychiatrist, are begging and convincing. Begging sounds like this:

"Please, please wear a mask. It will help protect your grandmother from getting COVID. I don't think she'd survive COVID if she got it."

There are very few people who won't be convinced to do something if you plead with them, beg them to do it.

Convincing appeals to a person's rational side and sounds like this:

"I know the precautions keep changing but can we figure out what makes sense for you and do it? We'll work out a good plan together."

While you are begging and convincing, do not worry if your emotions spill out. They should. You are, after all, worried that your child might get very sick – or even die. If your child accuses you of becoming dramatic, admit that you probably are. Admit that you love them too much for their difficulties and worries not to upset you deeply.

As someone who grew up in the comfortable 1970s, my life has been easier than that of the youth I work with. My generation of white people had the privilege to go to university on ample government loans and to go to work in comfortable jobs. We were untouched by world wars or economic depressions or pandemics. I often worry that I am not well-equipped to help young people through today's challenges.

I am so glad that youth are back in programs and in school. I missed my exasperating, infuriating, inspiring, and exhilarating teenage patients. I missed watching the shows they love with them, eating popcorn, playing pool, and baking cookies.

I missed their poetry and artwork where the wildness of youth is captured. Much of it was removed from the walls and the bulletin boards for their creators to take home when the pandemic started. Nothing captures the idealism of youth like poetry and artwork. Nothing captures the despair of youth like artwork and poetry.

Recent research from McGill University shows that the mental health impact of the pandemic was not as great as we had worried about.[4] Given all the stressors and changes experienced during the pandemic, this suggests that we were able to protect ourselves and our families from worse outcomes. Because of isolation, however, one mistake we made as a society was letting the pandemic interfere with the natural wildness of youth and their need to be with each other. We should never let the world tame our children.

DR. GAIL BECK is the Interim Chief of Staff and Clinical Director of Youth Mental Health at The Royal Ottawa Mental Health Centre in Ottawa, Canada. Her career has focused on championing the health needs of women and children.

The Pandemic Ends ... Then What?

ANNIE LIN

Summer 2021.

I am the sole, single parent to a disabled youth who has complex medical needs and multiple risk factors for severe or fatal effects from COVID-19. I have been parenting, homeschooling, and caregiving without any support or breaks for over fourteen months. My daughter is the sunshine in my days, but parenting someone with complex needs presents unique and exhausting challenges even during "normal" times, let alone with the added stress of a pandemic. Depleted doesn't even come close to describing the reality of my current state. I am done.

Over the years, one of my daughter's medical challenges has been significant struggles with her breathing – reactive airways/asthma, recurrent pneumonias, and respiratory distress. This has meant long-term heavy duty meds, including some that have decreased her immune system further, as well as many ER visits, multiple hospitalizations, and an outrageous amount of missed school. At its worst, she nearly died from influenza, needing to be resuscitated and put on a ventilator in the PICU of our local children's hospital.

Because of this, we have been supremely cautious and have lived on the extreme end of isolation during the pandemic: no indoor visits; only distanced outdoor visits with masks. We stopped all in-person speech and language therapy, physiotherapy, and occupational therapy; much of her medical care has been put on hold, and we've had delays to her medical imaging and surgeries. We have done no recreational or in-person educational activities. We have not gone inside a grocery store, eaten at a restaurant, or been inside the homes of any friends or family. We even limit playing at the park while other kids are there. Our only indoor interactions have been medical appointments. It is a constant calculation of risk, with any level of risk being taken only when absolutely and immediately necessary.

Some people think I've been overly restrictive – and I can understand their perspective – but when you've lived the life we have, that fear for your child's life never goes away. That risk of hospitalization and death lives under the surface of every decision, every interaction.

My daughter also has significant speech and language delays so she doesn't have the capacity for reciprocal conversation. Additionally, she has hearing loss and language processing delays, so virtual interactions are a big struggle and often end with her feeling more excluded. And because my life is tied directly to hers, this means I go days or weeks without actual conversation. The vast majority of my interactions during this pandemic have been virtual or by phone, but I struggle to interact meaningfully in this way and it generally leaves me more drained.

Truly, I have never felt so alone. My mental and physical health have suffered from the isolation and weight of worry. And my daughter has lost all meaningful opportunity for peer interaction. It has been impossibly and unimaginably hard.

And yet ...

I'm terrified for this pandemic to end. Not because I don't want the debilitating fears to go away, but because I don't know how we'll ever reintegrate back into society. My daughter is the most delightful person I've ever known and I'm angry and heartbroken over how people have refused to sacrifice any of their own privilege, or to advocate for or change their behaviours in the interest of those more vulnerable like her. Some of our own family and friends have chosen to remain unimmunized and many aren't wearing masks except when mandated. I don't know how to forget that. I don't know how to forgive. They have abandoned us, and left my daughter for dead.

I also had to leave my job early in the pandemic when it was all too much. I've lost the only reliable childcare provider I had. The friends I could rely on and relate to who are also parenting kids with disabilities and complex needs have moved away. So right now, I'm alone but under the guise of COVID. What happens when I don't have the pandemic to hide behind? We have lost everything.

The federal government has thankfully provided caregiver funding to families like mine during this time to stay afloat. But what happens when that ends? I have no job and no one to care for my daughter even if I did. We have no means or support to reintegrate. Who will step in to ensure we have the tools to survive? I fear no one will.

And then there is this: my daughter is thriving. While she misses her friends and activities and our regular trips to the doctors, the freedom she's been given to learn and play – to communicate and develop on her own terms – has been life-giving for her. The ability to move her body only if and when it feels good has meant a significant reduction in her chronic pain. And having just one adult to work with, as well as one stable and consistent routine, has allowed her language to grow. She is flourishing. What do I do with that? How are we supposed to move forward from here?

Post-pandemic life looks bleak from our vantage point. Who is planning for us? Or even just considering us? It feels impossible to look forward, to have hope for better. But I dream of a shift in society where people will actually care for the vulnerable around them. Where caregiving is recognized as the necessity that it is, with sufficient, ongoing, and accessible financial support. I long for a future where our systems aren't so embedded with ableism; where there is guidance from health and political leaders that not only specifically considers families like mine in planning but also centres our dignity and access needs. Then we wouldn't feel so abandoned, so alone. That is a hopeful future.

In post-pandemic life, that's what I long for: to be supported to integrate back into society in a way that works for us, where we can trust that it will be safe for us to not only live but also to thrive. My daughter deserves that. She needs that. And so do I. Do you see us? Will you plan for us?

ANNIE LIN is an independent, creative soul who loves being a mama. She is an RN by trade and a disability advocate. Gratitude, laughter, and her girl keep her centred.

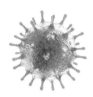

PART III

THE CRUMBLING BASE

Our healthcare system cannot function without the vital roles played by nurses, social workers, personal support workers, other allied healthcare professionals, and essential family caregivers. These roles are by and large, but not exclusively, filled by women. Their work is undervalued, rendered invisible, and taken for granted. Their importance – and vulnerability – was highlighted in the COVID-19 pandemic, as they became sick, burned out, and excluded from medical institutions. Yet they pushed back as strong advocates for their patients and communities. In this section, they implore us to listen to their powerful, important voices.

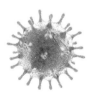

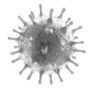

Resilience Is a Dirty Word

DEBRA LEFEBVRE

As my fellow nurse hung her head, exhausted, barely holding on, the manager passed by and glibly said, "Oh, come on. Where's your resilience?"

Resilience is a dirty word. Resilience is an overused word and it feels like it puts the systemic failings of the Ontario healthcare system squarely onto nurses' shoulders. The failings are many, including short staffing, underfunding, crowding, poor mental health resources, and violence and abuse, all of which break the backs and spirits of nurses. According to the Registered Nurses' Association of Ontario, even before the pandemic, Ontario had fewer beds per capita than the rest of Canada and we were short 22,000 nurses.[1] Nursing was breaking before COVID-19 hit.

The pandemic has only exacerbated the situation by causing a nursing shortage of crisis proportions due to nurses feeling disrespected, underpaid, overworked, and undervalued. Chronic trauma and stress have plagued nurses forever, but more so since the pandemic. In January 2021, at the height of the pandemic, a nurse died by suicide. I did not know her, but my colleagues and I grieved her death and its meaning. I'm sure some felt that she was not resilient enough. They would be wrong.

Despite being hailed as heroes, we felt abandoned and unsupported, and were fatigued and morally injured. How could we be resilient when faced with the overwhelming and persistent fear of caring for patients with insufficient personal protective equipment (PPE), unmanageable and unsafe workloads, the demands of navigating unfamiliar clinical settings as we were moved from one setting to another, and the lack of governmental and organizational support?

People do not realize that when healthcare is challenged, the burden to keep everything moving is on nurses. It is nurses who juggle larger workloads under extreme duress, not the government, nurse managers, or chief executive officers. We don't have time to think about being resilient.

Your Nurse Is Not OK

A pre-pandemic study conducted by the Canadian Federation of Nurses Unions (CFNU) revealed shocking levels of mental illness among nurses, only made worse during the pandemic.[2] Declining mental health continued unabated as we battled COVID-19. In a report by the CFNU in 2022, 94 per cent of nurses were showing signs of burnout, and

83 per cent said they were so understaffed that they worried about the quality of care they could provide.[3] Nurses were not only juggling multiple patients and numerous nursing interventions at the same time but were also providing emotional support to families as they said their final goodbyes to a loved one. Since the pandemic began, nurses were often the only ones to hold a dying patient's hand because of visitor restrictions, and even then, not as long as we may have wanted to because of workload and other patient demands. We will carry that burden for the rest of our lives.

According to the CFNU, rates of anxiety and depression in nurses have increased by 40 per cent since the pandemic began; our emotional pain can result in PTSD and burnout, which leads to even fewer nurses. It's not just practising nurses who suffer and lose their resilience; student nurses are affected, as well. In a meta-analysis conducted by Barrett and Twycross in 2022, the results show that one out of two nursing students suffers from depression.[4]

Instead of Resilience, Let's Talk about Moral Injury

As I write this, we are in the eighth wave of the pandemic and moral injury to nurses has greatly worsened. We find it extremely difficult to provide safe, quality care as a result of our workload. This is killing us. We are trained to care for our patients, and when we cannot because of forces beyond our control, we are morally injured. We feel betrayed and let down by government and healthcare leaders especially when we must fight for PPE, or when we feel a manager has not made every effort to backfill when we are short staffed.

What should terrify everyone is that nurses have been leaving the profession entirely since the beginning of the pandemic or they have been changing jobs. The 2022 CFNU survey showed that nearly half of the nurses who are currently working wish to change jobs due to job stress or concerns about mental health. A Statistics Canada Labour Force Survey released in June 2022 showed that 92 per cent of nurses said they were more stressed, and burnout was the most common reason why they planned to leave or change their jobs.[5] Reading between the lines, this means nurses working in increasingly high-stress areas, such as emergency, intensive care, and acute medicine, will leave these units to work elsewhere due to increased work demands and poor mental health and well-being because they worry about the quality of care they provide. The loss of experienced nurses will add more strain to an already collapsing healthcare system, and new nurses will have fewer veteran nurses to mentor them. Meanwhile, the nursing shortage is deepening and further eroding my ability to provide safe, quality care because my workload is growing. Nursing vacancies are more than triple (+219.8 per cent) the level that they were five years earlier, according to one study.[6]

Emotional fatigue can reduce cognitive functioning, including abilities such as decision-making, memory, and attention. When nurses are exhausted, things can be missed, and patient care can be compromised. In speaking with a physician the other day, I wondered aloud why we had not heard more about the occurrence of critical incidents. In a hushed voice, the physician remarked she was involved in a review where serious harm had occurred to a patient as a direct result of nurses being stretched too thin. Knowing the stress and duress that nurses are working under, this was unsurprising to us both. Forty-five emergency departments closed in 2022 because of extremely unsafe patient care, working conditions, and nursing shortages. Given the lack of a huge public outcry, I can only assume that Canadians are either oblivious, paralyzed, or resigned to the magnitude of the situation.

What also puzzles me is the harassment and bullying that occurs when nurses speak out. The nursing curriculum stresses repeatedly that patient advocacy is a significant role of the professional nurse. Yet when nurses speak out and stand up for safe, quality patient care, they are threatened, intimidated, and muzzled by their employers. The toxic culture of silencing is historic, pervasive, and entirely wrong. No nurse should feel threatened or silenced for advocating for the health of ALL Canadians, always and everywhere.

Violence and abuse also contribute to moral injury. A 2022 survey by the Canadian Union of Public Employees showed that physical violence on the job has been on the rise since the pandemic, and that it is very real and "part of the job" for nurses.[7] According to the CFNU's 2020 survey, physical assault was the most reported type of trauma exposure, affecting 92.7 per cent of nurses.[8] There have been times when I have been hit or kicked so hard that pain and deep bruising have resulted. There was a time when I was strangled by a patient and thought I would die. Sexual and verbal abuse is also on the rise, which started pre-pandemic. These incidents are demoralizing and demeaning and can affect our self-esteem. Despite hospital policies claiming "zero tolerance" towards violence and abuse, nurses must complete incident reports that ask us what we could have done differently to prevent the incident. We are the ones who mitigate these assaults and yet we do not receive supportive feedback or see any meaningful change in policy or procedure concerning violence and assault. Incident reporting seems hollow and a waste of time, and time is a luxury that we do not have.

All this and wage suppression, too. Introduced in 2019 by the Ontario government, Bill 124 limits wage increases to a maximum of 1 per cent per year for three years, suppressing a nurse's democratic right to negotiate for a higher salary. A recent court decision determined Bill 124 unconstitutional, and yet the Ontario government is appealing the decision and taking nurses to court. We view the government's challenge as another slap in the face, as well as a deep lack of respect for our profession.

The assault on nurses' well-being has been sustained over a long period of time, with no end in sight. Wave after wave of COVID-19 disease, illness, and death have washed over me and my colleagues, leaving us physically and emotionally exhausted, morally injured, and frustrated. Our resilience continues to be challenged amid this chaos, toxicity, and unhealthy workplace environments, and for many, our resilience wanes or is lost. Therefore, the next time a manager says the nasty words "dig deeper" or "find your resilience," please forgive us if we noticeably roll our eyes or a scream escapes.

We Are Done

Canada, and most certainly Ontario, is in a healthcare crisis. In Ontario, the nursing shortage is at an unprecedented level and should be on the minds of all Ontarians needing care. In Ontario alone, hospitals face a 20 per cent vacancy rate for nursing positions, according to the Ontario Nurses' Association.[9] According to a 2022 Canadian Institute for Health Information report, the Canadian average of registered nurses (RNs) per 100,000 citizens is 830.5. In Ontario, the average number of RNs per 100,000 people is just 668. Based on the report's data, Ontario would need to immediately hire more than 24,000 RNs to meet the national average.[10] That figure is up from 22,000 pre-pandemic and 17,000 a decade ago. Nurses are the backbone of healthcare, and our backs are broken. Morale is dangerously low, and crushing workloads and the level of despair and sadness is unprecedented. I have seen nurses with twenty-five years of experience leave my unit because of poor mental health; they could not tolerate the compromises made in patient care any longer nor the disrespect shown towards them. Nurses are the eyes and ears on a patient twenty-four hours a day, seven days a week. Nurses assess, monitor, interpret, and report changes in a patient's condition. We help soothe, heal, and save lives. When a patient is in need, the patient cries out, "NURSE. HELP ME!" We are the ones who are there first for the patient. When nurses are done, patient care is also done.

How You Can Help Nurses: Write to Your Provincial Government Official

The nursing crisis calls for urgent, coordinated, and multi-faceted actions by all levels of government and healthcare leaders. Nurses are sounding the alarm louder than ever before. If we don't act now to improve the retention, recruitment, and support of nurses, we risk a system-wide failure of our healthcare system.

1 Rates of anxiety and depression among nurses and nursing students have skyrocketed during the pandemic. We can surmise that the prolonged and sustained impact of the pandemic will only add to this trend. A call to timely compassionate action is needed to protect nursing students from the harmful effects of stress. Funding must be provided to Ontario's faculties of nursing for teaching nursing students emotional coping strategies to prepare them for professional practice. All nurses and nursing students also need guaranteed access to adequate and responsive mental health services. This solution should help the retention, recruitment, and support of nurses and future nurses. Write to your provincial government official.

2 All nurses deserve a safe, healthy, and supportive work environment. Employers must foster environments that

are free from violence and abuse. Research shows that unhealthy work environments have negative impacts on nurses, leading to poor patient care. As recommended by the House of Commons Standing Committee on Health in 2019, a national awareness campaign about violence against nurses and a prevention framework would be helpful. An increase in the number of security personnel in the work environment to respond to and protect nurses from violence and abuse is needed. This solution should help with the retention, recruitment, and support of nurses. Write to your provincial government official.

3 Legislated minimum nurse-to-patient ratio policies have demonstrated benefits in reducing nursing workloads, especially in acute care settings.[11] Extensive evidence shows that adopting safe nurse-patient ratios has significantly contributed to reducing crushing workloads, ensuring nurse safety and, thus, allowing patients to receive safe, quality care services. This solution should help the retention, recruitment, and support of nurses. Write to your provincial government official.

4 In Ontario, nurses must be exempt from Bill 124 to allow us to negotiate competitive compensation levels. Nurses' income, in real terms, has steadily declined by 20 per cent since 2010 as a result of Bill 124 and inflation. Nurses across Canada deserve to be better paid for the level of responsibility we have and the increase in the patient care workload. It is long overdue. In addition, if we are working short-handed, we should receive danger pay for the level of risk we endure. This solution should

help the retention, recruitment, and support of nurses. Write to your provincial government official.

5 There are approximately 20,000 internationally educated nurses living in Ontario and thousands more across Canada but they face numerous barriers to practise. Provincial nursing regulatory bodies must streamline and expedite the lengthy process of granting nursing licences to qualified and competent internationally educated nurses. This solution should help the retention, recruitment, and support of nurses. Write to your provincial government official.

6 Admissions to all nursing baccalaureate programs must be bolstered by 10 per cent in each of the next four years, and the supply of nurse practitioners must be increased by over 50 per cent by 2030. While the candidates will not graduate for at least four years, bolstering admissions to nursing baccalaureate programs will provide support for the future as we anticipate more nurses will leave patient care due to retirement or resignation. This solution should help the retention, recruitment, and support of nurses. Write to your provincial government official.

7 The recent appointments of chief nursing officers by the federal government and the Ontario government are welcome steps to bringing the voice of nursing to senior policymaking tables. The voice of nursing is needed in the development of standardized health data collection and analysis, as well as the development of systems that allow each jurisdiction to better manage and project health human resources in the future. This nursing

shortage crisis was avoidable. Hearing and respecting the voice of nursing will help to prevent it from happening again. Therefore, all provincial and territorial governments should have the voice of nursing at senior decision-making tables. This solution should help the retention, recruitment, and support of nurses. Write to your provincial government official.

For nearly three years, nurses have shouldered the enormous burden of the pandemic. We have no resilience left. We need your help.

DEBRA LEFEBVRE, RN, BN, BA, MPA, is an award-winning trauma-informed mental health nurse leader. She sits on the Board of Directors of the Registered Nurses' Association of Ontario. She is the owner of Limestone City Mental Health, a wellness agency focused on individual and workplace mental health. Debra is also the co-founder of ThriveAbility, an agency that helps people and organizations transform and restore strength, build connections, improve mental health, and increase productivity through storytelling and education.

Men Write the Policies, Women Face the Results

DR. MICHELLE COHEN

I sit here contemplating how much more I can take and give of myself. Years being a nurse, I used to be happy, vigilant, and ready to face it all. This pandemic has not only made me depressed and anxious but cold. Cold to the patients, as I get hit, punched and screamed at. Cold to my own compassion. Am I punishing myself staying in a field that has no more gratitude? From denied time off, no vacation, reusing N95's. Short staffed. Healthcare Hero's my ass. Underpaid and continued to be abused. Yet. Here we are still showing up. The punishment of a nurse.

                              – Anonymous entry to MyCovidStory.ca (2022)[1]

Imagine for a moment it's 2019 and you're sitting at home reading the newly released World Health Organization (WHO) report called *Delivered by Women, Led by Men*. The report lays out the gender dynamics of a global health sector where women dominate by numbers yet are seg-regated into lower paid, lower status, less safe jobs.[2] (See Figure 16.1.) Suddenly a time traveller from the future materializes with an urgent warning: In one year, a novel respiratory virus will tear across the planet, the impact of which will be unlike any other infectious disease in re-corded history. How would you foresee this tidal wave of illness affecting the female-dominated but male-led health sector?

Globally, 70 per cent of the health workforce's[3] front-line services are provided by women,[4] but in Canada this proportion is over 80 per cent.[5] This can be interpreted as a relatively high number of women in Canadian medicine; however, health leadership, the administrative level where the sector's policies are written, is still a space women have a hard time entering.[6] Most women working in the Cana-dian health sector do lower-paying front-line care work such as nursing or personal support work (PSW), both of which are over 90 per cent female.[7] Health policy on the whole is written by men and carried out by women, which is a fact rarely considered in the crafting of such policies.

Learning from Canadian Statistics

The term [is] compassion exploitation … look how many women work in healthcare … society has fostered that women are compas-sionate. They have created this, and I do think that it is definitely being exploited during the pandemic.

– Community Health Worker, quoted in *Invisible No More*[8]

FIGURE 16.1. *Global health leadership pyramid. Women's representation in global health leadership, based on influence. Graphic from* **Delivered by Women, Led by Men** *(WHO, 2019).*

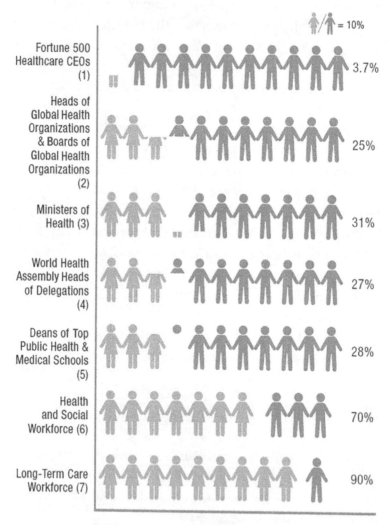

They call us guardian angels, but they treat us like numbers. I'm immunocompromised and failing my fourth treatment for multiple sclerosis. They are refusing my neurologist's medical note and denying my leave. I'm a guardian angel, so I have to continue working despite his advice. I'm a nurse, but I'm seen as a guardian angel.

– Nurse, quoted in "Blowing the Whistle"[9]

Global Health 50/50 is a research and advocacy initiative for gender equity that has created a publicly available tool called the "COVID-19 Sex-Disaggregated Data Tracker."[10] The Tracker was updated regularly from 2020 to 2022, the years when countries openly reported their COVID-19 statistics. Of the forty-two countries that collected sex-disaggregated COVID-19 data on health workers, Canada ranked ninth highest in the female proportion of cases. Among the ten Organisation for Economic Co-operation and Development (OECD) member countries in that group, Canada had the second most feminized COVID-19 case burden among health workers (Figure 16.2), a ratio similar to the ratio of women in front-line heath work.

Throughout 2020, health workers shouldered a high burden of infection, making up nearly one in ten of all documented COVID-19 cases that year, which is unsurprising given high case counts in long-term care (LTC) facilities and the resulting toll on hospitals and other health facilities.[11] The LTC sector fared particularly poorly in the pre-vaccine era, with LTC residents suffering 69 per cent of all COVID-19 deaths prior to March 2021, a substantially higher proportion than the international average of 41 per cent.[12]

The gender breakdown among LTC residents is roughly two-thirds female, which is why the industry is sometimes

FIGURE 16.2. *COVID-19 cases in health workers by gender. Cases in health workers among OECD nations that track sex-disaggregated COVID-19 data, April 2020–July 2022.*

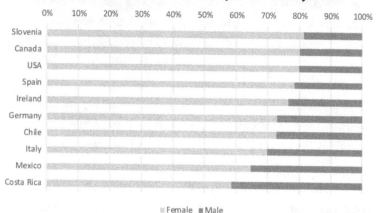

From The Sex, Gender and COVID-19 Project, "Sex-Disaggregated Data Tracker"

described as women workers caring for mostly women clients. Many experts feel these gender statistics explain the sector's low status and dearth of resources.[13] The COVID-19 devastation in Canadian LTC homes made a gendered impact on early pandemic mortality data. Globally, among the 140 countries that collected sex-disaggregated COVID-19 data, the ratio of male to female deaths was 1.3 as of mid-2022, meaning a higher mortality for men (13 male deaths for every 10 female deaths, or male deaths were 1.3 times higher than female deaths). Canadian COVID-19 data from mid-2022 show a male to female mortality ratio of 1.1 (Figure 16.3). However, prior to June 2021, mortality skewed female, averaging a ratio of 0.87 male to female from May 2020 until the end of that year.[14]

The feminized mortality of Canada's pre-vaccine COVID-19 era was thought to be a result of high rates of

FIGURE 16.3. *COVID-19 mortality in Canada by gender, April 2020 to August 2022.*

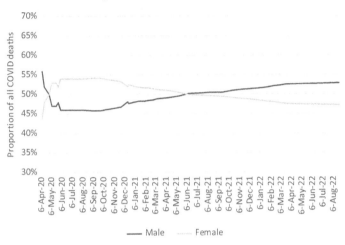

From The Sex, Gender and COVID-19 Project, "Sex-Disaggregated Data Tracker"

illness in LTC facilities.[15] However, data collected after widespread vaccinations suggest that overall workplace risk continued to be feminized, even though mortality had declined. While men comprised nearly 53 per cent of COVID-19 deaths by mid-2022, they made up only 46 per cent of cases.[16] Disaggregating data further by age shows higher case counts for women of working age (Figure 16.4). This is concordant with Canadian data showing that health workers with COVID-19 tended to be female and younger than the general population.[17] Women also tended to have higher vaccination rates as a group, which may reflect workplace policies on vaccination and would be expected to decrease the likelihood of mortality.[18] Taken together these statistics indicate a gender difference in the risk of contracting COVID-19 in the workplace.

FIGURE 16.4. *COVID-19 cases (top) and mortality (bottom) by age and gender in Canada, April 2020 to July 2022 (rates per 100,000).*

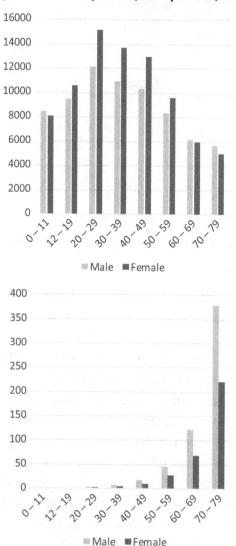

From *The Sex, Gender and COVID-19 Project*, "*Sex-Disaggregated Data Tracker*"

More research is needed to better understand these disparities, but it is not unreasonable to theorize that the gender dynamics of the health workforce are a contributing factor to higher rates of infection among working age women in Canada.

Learning from Health Worker Stories

I was willing and able to go to work in that completely broken state because I'm a nurse and that's what nurses do.

– Nurse, quoted in "The Experiences of Nurses in British Columbia"[19]

I have a lot of friends still working in LTC, and they're struggling. They're overworked and underpaid, and the facilities are terribly understaffed. The public doesn't hear much about what goes on inside for-profit facilities because workers tend to stay tight-lipped for fear of losing their jobs.

– Tina James, PSW[20]

Tina James had been a PSW in Toronto for nine years when she caught COVID-19 in May of 2020, only two weeks after she started a new job in an LTC facility. In a January 2021 article for *Toronto Life*, she recalls feeling fearful because of how unknown COVID-19 was at the time. She worried about the implications for her elderly mother, gathering her family together over a video call to plan for her mother's care should Tina wind up in the hospital. She was ill for weeks, too tired at times to shower without her partner's help. When her acute symptoms abated after one month, Tina returned to a traumatized workplace:

> I was still testing positive, but because I was no longer symp-
> tomatic, my supervisor said that I had to go back to work. By
> the time I got there, the mood was eerie. Ten more residents
> had died from Covid while I was gone. A few PSWs on my
> floor had tested positive at the same time that I did, so some
> of them were still off, and there were a lot of new workers in
> the building.[21]

Tina's return to work was marred by long COVID symptoms like shortness of breath, persistent cough, and brain
fog. In September of 2020, she realized that she could no
longer work in LTC. Leaving her job made her feel sad but
also gave her a sense of relief. She left behind a battered industry, one that still was endangering her friends, many of
whom fell ill and one who has died.

> A lot of PSWs stopped showing up for work because they
> were scared, or because they had been exposed to a resident
> who had Covid and needed to isolate at home. The facility
> tried to fill those vacancies by calling in casual employees
> or going through agencies. The staff was changing over a
> lot, but we were still always short-staffed, and that put more
> pressure on the people who did show up for work.[22]

In Ontario's LTC facilities, PSWs comprise 58 per cent
of all employees, followed by registered nurses (RNs) at
25 per cent.[23] This means the principal employee in the

LTC sector is an unregulated class of health worker who works without a union or a negotiating body. PSWs can be considered precarious workers, defined as employees without job security or promotion opportunities who typically earn low wages with no benefits in unregulated or unsafe conditions.[24]

Many aspects of PSWs' precarity increase the risk of COVID-19 infection. As health workers, PSWs are often afforded poor access to personal protective equipment (PPE), despite working on the front lines of the worst outbreaks.[25] Working in multiple facilities because of poor job security increases the likelihood of COVID-19 transmission between facilities;[26] the lack of benefits coupled with little-to-no sick leave further erodes safety, as many PSWs feel they have no option but to go to work sick.

Susan, a pseudonymous PSW interviewed on the CBC Radio show *White Coat, Black Art* in May of 2020, said her LTC facility was so severely short-staffed that she felt "obliged" to return to work, despite ongoing COVID-19 symptoms. As both case counts and deaths continued to climb at her facility, she worried about her possible role in the outbreak: "I can't help but sit there and look back, you know, did I infect any of my co-workers or did I infect any of my residents? Am I going to have to see them get sick? Am I going to have to see any of them die? And think, it could have been my fault. It's just very distressing."[27]

In addition to being overwhelmingly female, PSWs are a highly racialized group, with over 40 per cent of PSWs on a recent survey identifying as a visible minority.[28] The proportion of PSWs in Canada who are migrants increased from 22 per cent to 36 per cent between 1996 and 2016, reflecting similar trends in care work in other countries of the Global North.[29] As a group, migrants are over-represented in the front-line health workforce[30] and this is especially true in urban areas, with a recent survey of 664 PSWs in Toronto showing that over 97 per cent were born outside Canada.[31] The number of migrant health workers in the Canadian LTC sector has been growing for many years, and in some provinces, half of LTC health workers are migrants.[32]

Despite the recency of these data, migrant care labour in Canada has a long history, dating back to early twentieth-century immigration programs aimed at Caribbean women. Such programs later evolved into the recruitment of Filipina women, and today both groups are concentrated in care work.[33] The low status of PSWs in the Canadian health sector cannot be separated from the over-representation of racialized and migrant women within their ranks.

The broader COVID-19 data demonstrate greater risk associated with racialized status and lower income, in large part due to higher rates of precarious work in congregant settings such as factories, warehouses, and farms.[34] Narrowing the focus to the health sector reveals the risk to be deeply structural along similar lines of precarity. The least protected workers are lower-paid women, often racialized and from groups who have historically been occupationally segregated into migrant care work. Understanding the pandemic's impact on the health sector requires knowledge of how risk in health work is structurally gendered and racialized.

Women's Many Care Roles

The biggest thing at the very beginning for myself was my child-care for my dependents ... I basically had to take 50% of my job off to care for them because, at least in our community, THERE IS AN ABSOLUTE CHILDCARE CRISIS ALREADY. And Covid made that so much worse.

– Community Health Worker, quoted in *Invisible No More*[35]

My kids had to isolate and were sent home. The school calls me at one pm and assumes that I should just go home and take care of the kids, even though my husband is far more flexible with his schedule. Why didn't they call him?

– Physician, quoted in "I May Be Essential"[36]

The feminized burden of the pandemic and the resulting negative progress for women in the workplace has been described by many sources.[37] Owing to the disproportionate share of domestic responsibilities shouldered by women, school lockdowns and reductions in childcare and extra-curricular activities had a highly gendered impact. This is no less true of health workers. A 2021 study of female physicians in British Columbia found they faced unique challenges during the pandemic because of increased unpaid care responsibilities and the stress of maintaining the invisible barrier between the health workplace and home environment.[38] I can relate to these findings personally as a family physician with three school-aged children. Many women in the study reported feeling unable to juggle the additional demands that were disproportionately placed on them compared to male colleagues.

Infectious disease experts have studied and debated the possibility that children might be a viral reservoir for SARS-CoV-2, a way for viruses to spread undetected and thus never disappear.[39] Whether or not this has any real significance in the COVID-19 pandemic, it certainly raises a more general concern for a health workforce that is mostly female. As long as our society expects women to be the primary caregivers of children, the health workforce as a whole will be vulnerable to any pathogen that excels at spreading in classrooms and daycares.

Women also disproportionately do more unpaid care work for elders and loved ones with disabilities.[40] Commonly, those with special medical needs are also at higher risk from COVID-19. This can be an additional stressor for women in healthcare, who often carry the mental burden of worry (or guilt) about being an infectious vector for a loved one at higher risk.[41]

Multigenerational homes with larger families are thought to be one of many contributing factors to the higher COVID-19 burden in lower-income neighbourhoods.[42] Depending on the neighbourhood, many of the women living in low-income, multigenerational homes may be front-line health workers – and many of them are also likely doing some form of unpaid care work at home.

It bears considering from a health system sustainability perspective how wise it is for the bulk of labour to be performed by lower-paid, often precariously employed women. This is an especially salient discussion given all that we have come to understand about SARS-CoV-2's ability to exploit social inequities. In the added domestic and care loads that women bear, and in the inequitable structures that entrench poverty and racism, comes further COVID-19 risk for nearly all of the front-line health workforce.

Health Leaders in the Media

Male leaders were making decisions, that had to be made quickly, but also had a stay-at-home wife, or children who were no longer dependent on them.

– Physician, quoted in "I May Be Essential"[43]

We're healthcare heroes, but no. We're not actually treated as heroes by our actual employer. Not like you want to be treated like a hero … [but] we don't even have access to free coffee and tea, or a fridge.

– Nurse, quoted in "The Experiences of Nurses in British Columbia"[44]

Considering the gender breakdown of the Canadian health workforce and the at times all-consuming nature of COVID-19 news coverage, one would expect to see women health experts frequently in the media. Research on gender representation in Canadian news reporting has documented a slow increase in quotes from female sources from 17 per cent in 1995 to 24 per cent in 2015.[45] In data collected by the Gender Gap Tracker, a project associated with Simon Fraser University, the pandemic coincided with an uptick in quotes from female sources, which in late 2020 was reported as 31 per cent.[46]

The explosion in health-focused news has likely contributed to the increase in female representation in news media. Yet quotes from health worker sources do not reflect the gender breakdown of the health sector. In the three-year period between late 2018 and late 2021, the Gender Gap Tracker documented nearly 35,000 quotes in news media from health workers, 62 per cent of which were from women.[47] This is substantially lower than the over 80 per cent female representation in the Canadian health sector, suggesting that male health workers have a disproportionately larger presence on the public stage.

Media has long had a bias towards interviewing doctors over nurses or other health workers,[48] and at a time when so much focus was on intensive care units, the fact that more than three-quarters of (adult) intensivists[49] are men may have influenced gender representation in news reporting. And yet two other medical specialties often featured in the COVID-19 press, public health and infectious disease, are nearly at par between the binary genders.[50] The pandemic era's profuse flow of news stories about hospitals, LTC facilities, and high-risk health work did increase the visibility of non-physician front-line workers, but this was also largely due to skilful use of social media by health workers to gain attention and advocate for themselves, their colleagues, and their communities.[51]

One would expect the media to spend considerable time speaking to people in health leadership during a pandemic. Despite the movement of women into higher-status roles in the health sector, leadership has proved much slower to diversify its historical white and male dominance.[52] This is relevant on two fronts: first, health leadership is very removed from the lived experiences of the bulk of the health workforce; and second, the media amplifies a group disconnected from the front-line health worker, which in turn only reinforces to the public (and consequently the leadership) that front-line voices are not needed to flesh out the narrative of the pandemic.

Lack of representation in media narratives diminishes the visibility of risks to the front-line health workforce, and the knock-on effect of minimizing harms experienced by the less visible workforce is the continued reinforcement of those harms.

Thinking Back to 2019

As nurses, we're so good at compartmentalizing ... You see a lot of traumatic things, you sometimes are dealing with patients that are just in the aftermath of trauma and you got to put that in a box or in a room inside your mind and that's your work box, right? And when your home life is out of kilter and you don't have your support people, you don't have things to put back into your emotional bank, then you start to run on empty and then you take Benadryl and wine and hope that everything goes away.

– Nurse, quoted in "The Experiences of Nurses in British Columbia"[53]

Returning to our thought experiment: it's 2019 and you show *Delivered by Women, Led by Men* to your time-travelling visitor. The traveller tells you the PSW workforce was hit hard by the pandemic, alongside RNs and other lower status front-line health workers who are mainly female and often racialized.[54]

You and the traveller wonder how desegregating the health leadership pyramid in Figure 16.1 might have reduced the COVID-19 harms experienced by front-line health workers. Would access to PPE have been better, particularly in the early months of the pandemic when Canadian LTC facilities were supply-strapped but carried a high burden of infection? Would job precarity and the risks of PSWs working in multiple facilities have been more visible to health policymakers? Would we blithely expect mothers and caregivers to bear a sudden additional load while simultaneously calling on a mainly female workforce to protect the public from an infectious onslaught?

In a crisis where the burdens of public health restrictions fall heavily on women, it matters that the leadership writing policy is so very male so much of the time. Likewise it matters that job precarity and migration are experienced so rarely in the group that writes LTC policies. As one nurse recalls, she received the following note from her supervisor: "If you have to go off of work because you might be positive for COVID, we're not going to pay you for that either. It's going to come out of your sick [leave] or you get unpaid leave. So sorry about your luck."[55]

Imagine leaving 2019 and entering the COVID-19 era with policies sensitive to the realities at the bottom of the health leadership pyramid. This could mean better job security, better family leave and sick leave policies, more accessible childcare, better pay equity, and higher remunerative valuation of care labour in general. A more stable and better protected front-line workforce could have formed a stronger societal barrier against the pandemic, blunting its wider damage.

We can use our knowledge of COVID-19's gendered impact on the health sector to plan for a better outcome for the next health crisis humanity will face. Whether sparked by an infectious pathogen, climate change, or geopolitical instability, regional and global health crises are regular events in the history of our species and can be expected to continue in the future. We must evolve towards policies that fully grasp our segregated health workforce if we want to weather the next crisis more safely and equitably. Desegregating the health sector is also a goal to strive towards as part of the greater aim of a more equitable society. Careful feminist analysis of the impact of COVID-19 on the health workforce will better prepare us for the next health crisis and bolster our safety in the uncertain times ahead.

MICHELLE COHEN, MD, CCFP, FCFP, is a rural family physician and assistant professor in the Department of Family Medicine at Queen's University.

#InItTogether Is Only a Hashtag for Canadian Caregivers

MAGGIE KERESTECI

The much-loved Mr. Rogers of *Mr. Rogers' Neighborhood* used to tell us to "look for the helpers," and I often think of the many caregivers I speak to every day as the kind of helpers he was referring to. Most caregivers change their lives, alter their careers, balance responsibilities, and adapt goals to care for those who need them.

Well, right now the helpers need help. We are tired. We are stretched beyond imagining. COVID-19 did not cause the crisis for caregivers in Canada; it did make the crisis even more pressing.

I care for my octogenarian mother who lives with me, and I care for a relative with two cancers, one of which is a rare, insidious, and life-altering disease. They both depend on me for the mundane everyday needs of life, as well as the provision of complex medical support. They depend on me for navigation of a complex and disjointed health and social service system. They depend on me for emotional support. They depend on me to protect them from harm and to ensure they are cared for, not on an episodic basis, but 24/7.

During COVID-19, this has meant vigilance on every front, staying home for three years, seeking out and taking sound public health advice, and having to withstand the abuse and taunting of those who feel their "freedom" trumps the needs of community. I am also the sole breadwinner in my home. Like many caregivers, I have had to adjust my work responsibilities so that I can provide the care my family needs. It's safe to say that I feel stretched at the best of times. I fear that I am not performing any of these roles well or fully and that I am often the weakest link.

Throughout the pandemic, I have lived in fear of getting COVID because I know how many people depend on me for all aspects of life. The unimaginable happened just ten days after provincial restrictions were lifted: I had a high fever, blinding headache, and a chest-wracking cough. Eight of us in my family got sick and for me, the caregiver for my relatives, the consequences that played out were harrowing. The weight of responsibility and guilt that comes with being a caregiver who contracts an illness that could harm the people you care for is overwhelming. I was isolated at home with them and very afraid.

Many people have no idea of the deep-seated terror that you experience when you have done all that you could to protect the people you care for from illness, but you fail despite all your efforts. The fear that they will not survive or that, because you are sick, they will not be looked after is constant. Any time I get sick, or if I require hospitalization,

or succumb to an illness, the people I care for are left de-
fenceless and often fall through the cracks in our breaking healthcare system. There is no one to get groceries or
medicine, to prepare meals, or to give meds.

As a caregiver, I am the "project manager," so my having
COVID-19 meant several cancelled and rescheduled medical appointments that I had to organize in the midst of the
virus tearing through our home. It also meant that no one
else could come in to help me provide for their needs, and
there was certainly no one to care for me as I fought the virus. We existed on tea, water, juice, and a couple of cans of
soup that were in the cupboard. A neighbour dropped off
necessary medications, medical supplies, and kindly left a
casserole on my porch.

The infectiousness of COVID-19 meant there was no help
available, and we were left to manage by ourselves. One
morning, feverish with a staggering headache that left me
sleepless, I went to bring my eighty-eight-year-old mother
some tea. I found her in the bathroom on the floor, squeezed
between the sink and wall, unable to get up, drained of all
colour except for an ash grey pallor, in tears, and groaning
in pain. She did not know how long she had been there or
how she got there. She is nearly six feet tall and was im-
movable. The two of us struggled for hours. I eventually
found a way to move her, but it was painful for both of us.
I finally got her out of the confines of the bathroom, then
it took more than an hour to slide her back into her room
along the floor. Somehow, I lifted her into bed.

At the outset of the pandemic, as Canada scrambled to
prepare for the daily and exponential increases in COVID-19

cases, leaders across the system failed to consider family caregiving as a key component of our overall healthcare system planning. What has kept me going through this ordeal has not been government policies, programs, or legislation, but rather a community of allies. What has kept me going is finding my people, my circle of support, a caregiver and healthcare community of others willing to take a risk and speak up about the crisis in caregiving across Canada.

Being a family caregiver has always been an extremely isolating experience, even in the "before times." It's no surprise that our physical and mental health is suffering. In 2018 there were an estimated 7.8 million people providing care for family, friends, and neighbours in Canada.[1] Five years later that number is likely considerably higher given that there are now more than 8 million unpaid caregivers in Canada. Think for a moment of the impact on 8 million Canadians and those they care for.

Eight million of us who save the health system billions of dollars a year. Eight million of us who provide vital care that the system cannot or will not support. Eight million of us with stories not unlike mine. Eight million of us left to fend for ourselves during the worst public health crisis faced by this generation. Eight million of us who are not okay.[2]

There are millions of stories like mine. They prove that the state of caregiving today is not sustainable. If you take away the top stones from a pyramid nothing will happen. If, however, you weaken the bottom stones, the whole structure eventually crumbles and caves in. Caregivers are the bottom stones in the health system pyramid, and we are crumbling.

We need real system change with a national formal recognition of essential caregivers, with a common understanding of what caregiving means and the provision of formalized support. We need supports and regulations for the 35 per cent of the Canadian workforce who provide care while employed.[3] I am an active advocate and am familiar with navigating our complex system, but there has been virtually no support that I could access during COVID-19. It is urgent that Canada simplifies and coordinates a caregiver support system that moves us away from the highly fragmented and inaccessible system that exists today.

Caregivers do not have the time or the energy to seek out information and supports from multiple places, so it is essential that we create networks and resources that are readily available and are provided to caregivers by primary care, hospitals, and community agencies. Centralized information and resources mean that caregivers don't have to go searching for piecemeal help and so organizations such as the newly formed Canadian Centre for Caregiving Excellence can be of real help.[4] Caregivers benefit tremendously from peer support, from those who have shared the experience of caregiving. If hospitals and community agencies kept a registry of caregivers willing to support caregivers in the community who need it, that would be a tremendous win. Another support that is missing is education: education about the system and how to navigate it, education about a specific disease or condition and how to care for those with it, and education about how to advocate for care and change. These are just a few examples. There are countless ways to better support caregivers, and many of them are not sophisticated or expensive to implement. Ask a caregiver – they will tell you what is needed.

We need answers to some important and hard questions: What happens when the caregiver falls ill? Where is the support? How do we continue to care for our loved ones? Who will help the caregiver? We have been shouting our concerns for years with many heads nodding in agreement but no real change. The pandemic has revealed how fragile our system is and how undervalued and unsupported Canada's caregivers are and that, in fact, we are not #InItTogether.

We need to create a system that is centred on people and community and that recognizes the unique roles we each play in the well-being of others. I remain optimistic and will persevere in attempts to achieve a new reality for Canadian caregivers. My hope is for a future where caregivers are never again forgotten, where we get the support we need to thrive, not simply survive.

MAGGIE KERESTECI is an essential caregiver who advocates with caregivers across all sectors of the Canadian health system to support co-design of patient- and caregiver-inspired policies and programs. She is executive director at the Canadian Association for Health Services and Policy Research. She lives in rural southwestern Ontario.

Invisible

SARAH KAPLAN

In a moment, anyone can become a caregiver. Five years ago, I was walking with my husband when he collapsed. At that very moment, I became a full-time caregiver. Caregivers can be family, a spouse, neighbours, and friends.

Caregiving is on a continuum from supervisory to intermittent to full-time care of another person(s). Many caregivers also work for a living. A caregiver may find themselves thrown from a balanced life where they feel in control to one where they suddenly find themselves crazy busy with no private time. Friends disappear, social lives are disrupted, there is little time to look after their own health, and time to oneself becomes a luxury item.

When someone becomes a caregiver, there is often a learning curve. They need to learn about a potentially new illness that involves medications. They must liaise with different specialists. Their loved one may follow a restrictive diet. In our situation, the changes came within twenty-four hours, planting the seeds for years of serious mental health issues on my part.

Caregivers coordinate all health-related tasks such as medical appointments, blood tests, medication management, exercise, and social activities. They are the point of contact for banks, insurance companies, and homecare. Caregivers are the main mode of transportation to appointments and are often present at doctor appointments to take notes and carry out the duties of the care plan.

Caregivers oversee the duties in their loved one's home and may have to complete all of them all the time.

My daily agenda is one without reprieve from the caregiving role. Even at work in our local hospital, I received calls regarding the care of my husband. This caused me to be in a constant state of worry that my employer would think the quality of my work had declined or that I would be fired.

When I became a caregiver, I had to navigate complex systems, advocate endlessly, and fill in the gaps due to a lack of resources. Over time, this constant demand depleted my energy causing me to burn out. In addition to the stress from caregiving, the constant worry, fear, and feelings of helplessness contributed to a diagnosis of post-traumatic stress disorder (PTSD). Caregivers suffering from PTSD assert that they did not get this from one single traumatic event. The multitude of tasks, unkind interactions, navigating complex systems, and lack of support creates an environment conducive to the development of PTSD.

When being a caregiver was barely manageable for me, the pandemic hit. Very quickly, I lost my treasured six and a half hours of weekly homecare, my husband's transportation service to dialysis, and other informal supports. Due to the complexities of my husband's health, he could not be home alone and I had been redeployed and had to be in the hospital full time. Luckily, I was able to have my daughters take turns helping out but it was not ideal. But it wasn't ideal for anyone.

As the pandemic continued, my daughters had to return to their lives. Services were resurrected slowly. I went back to my position and then my husband got a kidney transplant. This was another fight. There was no understanding that he also had a brain injury to be accounted for and he needed me there to advocate for him.

The gift of a transplant comes with other concerns due to the immunosuppressant medication. While COVID-19 was the central worry, he was at increased risk for other infections. My role as caregiver was one of protector. The isolation that came with keeping him safe also contributed to my increasing mental health challenges. Every day, I lived with unbearable anxiety, long periods of depression, insomnia, obsession with his death and my own. Who would take care of him if something happened to me? I developed the COVID-19 fears. Every sniffle or cough he had sent tremors through my body.

While caregiving in itself has unique challenges and is extremely hard physically and emotionally, there are changes in healthcare that could improve the reality of caregivers.

The pandemic highlighted what most caregivers already know: the healthcare system needs to have a better understanding of their reality. The role of the caregiver is underappreciated. A patient can have a very complex medical history and require many specialists in the hospital, and yet this same patient is discharged to a caregiver who usually has no medical knowledge at all. The caregiver is informally coerced into being the care manager, coordinating all the information among specialists because once the patient is discharged, these professionals don't consult each other as frequently. Caregivers are rarely provided with adequate education and support to address the complexity that they face caring for their loved ones. They are an unacknowledged key player in patient care.

Caregiver inclusion has been a key strategic challenge that preceded the COVID-19 pandemic. During the pandemic, it came under the spotlight with respect to long-term care. Caregivers were quickly restricted from supporting their loved ones in healthcare facilities. The images of residents pressed against their windows just to get a glimpse of their loved ones outside was heartbreaking. We need to do better.

Including caregivers as part of the healthcare team is an undeniable return on investment. When caregivers are involved in healthcare, patient outcomes are improved. Caregiver involvement saves time for hospital staff. Working relationships between caregivers and healthcare professionals are critical to the quality of care for the patient. Caregivers will often be the ones ensuring that the care plan and other medical guidelines are followed. They make sure that appointments are attended. Caregivers will research and educate themselves on how best to take care of their loved ones. The current state is that caregivers and healthcare professionals work in silos while both are working for the patient. Working together is the best use of their respective expertise. It saves time and money and creates the best opportunity for improved outcomes for the patients. Caregiver wellness also improves when their role is respected, and they are included.

A couple of months ago, we had an appointment with a new doctor. This always worries me because usually I must repeat the story of why I am involved and why I am at this appointment and why I do much of the talking. The doctor greeted us both by name. He never once questioned why I was there and treated me through words and gestures as a respected member of the team. He asked how I was doing. He asked if I needed anything. He reviewed all the decisions at the end and clearly stated what I was to do and what he would do. He did all of this with a deep respect for both of us, and he was very kind. So simple. My husband and I left the appointment happy. We felt heard. He validated my experience simply by acknowledging my role. It was clear to me that he understood the health impact of caregiving.

The health of the caregiver must be considered in the overall health of the patient. This doesn't mean that when a healthcare professional cares for a patient they need to take care of the caregiver as well. What is important is to assess how the caregiver is doing and acknowledge their reality and refer them to an appropriate resource. If this is done sincerely and with kindness, perhaps more caregivers would not be unwell. It has to be more than the cliché of "don't forget to take care of yourself."

A caregiver who is supported will use the system less for themselves. Due to my mental health issues, I became a patient and used many services for my physical and mental health. I believe that had I been supported, included, and respected, there would not have been such a dramatic impact to my health.

Decisions can be made to include caregivers in a few important ways:

- With patient consent, document the contact information of the caregiver.
- After each intervention/treatment, ensure the caregiver is updated.
- Routinely ask about the caregiver (example questions):
    - How is your physical and mental health? Are you sleeping? Do you feel anxious at times? Do you have time to yourself? Does anyone help you in your role? Do you have interests/hobbies of your own?
    - Is there anything you need to help you in your caregiving role? Do you have homecare?
- If appropriate, refer to a social worker to complete a caregiver stress assessment and to provide support/referrals.
- Include caregivers in discharge planning.

Here are a few points that helped me on my caregiving journey:

1 My #1 rule is to protect yourself:
    - When possible, don't always give up your important time for appointments for your loved one.
    - Book appointments at times that are good for you and, when possible, do not have too many in the same day or with a lot of driving.
    - Ensure time for meals, exercise, and down time.
    - Find homecare or activities for your loved one so you can have time to yourself.

o Find meaning in your own work, hobbies,
   activities: you are more than a caregiver.
2 Take the time and make the effort to build relationships
   with everyone involved in the care team from clerks
   to doctors, from the homecare supervisor to your case
   manager for long-term disability or contact at your
   insurance company.
3 Keep good notes on your loved one's medical information. I use an iPad and have it on hand when my husband is admitted to the hospital and at all appointments.
4 Learn to love technology. Medical records are accessible
   electronically from most hospitals and labs. This way
   you can keep up with important results.
5 Notes
   o We have "before going to a medical appointment"
      notes so we don't forget important information at
      an appointment.
6 Practise being assertive about your role. Do not apologize for asking the healthcare professional a question.
   You are helping them in their job. When your loved
   one is in the hospital, you are more than just a visitor. If
   you want your important role to be respected, then you
   need to expect the respect.
   o Try as best you can to communicate well even
      when the subject matter is difficult.
   o State the facts and don't leave until you have a plan.
   o Educate yourself on your rights; for example, dur-
      ing COVID-19, I knew that legally, I was allowed to
      accompany my husband when he was hospitalized
      due to his brain injury. Many hospital staff were un-
      aware. Learn about policies/laws that impact you.

7 As soon as you notice a few weeks of insomnia, anxiety, new physical pain, or other health issues that seem odd, don't wait, see someone soon and take care of your health. You are doing this not only so you can take care of another, you are doing this because you deserve to be well. Caregiving is a risk to mental and physical health, so do a check up on yourself.

8 When you are ready, you might benefit from a caregiver support group

9 Ask someone for help to:
   o Sit with your loved one for two hours
   o Buy groceries
   o Make a meal
   o Provide transportation
   o Pick up medications

10 Helpful websites:
   o Canadian Centre for Caregiving Excellence, https://canadiancaregiving.org/
   o The Ontario Caregiver Organization, https://ontariocaregiver.ca/

Pandemic or no pandemic, it will benefit all healthcare organizations to create caregiver inclusive policies to improve the overall health of both patients and their caregivers.

SARAH KAPLAN, MSW (retired), is a retired social worker. She previously managed a medical forensic program and led change projects, focusing on caregiver inclusion in healthcare, new mental health programs, and community strategic alliances. She currently writes about the health impact of caregiving with special interest in post-traumatic stress disorder.

The Levee Has Broken

KIM ENGLISH

During the early years of the pandemic, we heard the pots and pans banging in appreciation, saw the signs and hearts in windows, and watched the drive-bys and listened to the accolades calling nurses healthcare heroes. Now, the banging in appreciation has been replaced by the drumming of threats and hate. And the silence of a society that no longer cares or, worse, blames and questions nurses and other healthcare providers.

The Doug Ford government in Ontario, re-elected in 2022 with a majority government, has been devastating for nurses. The decision to implement Bills 195 and 124, effectively restricting wage increases for public sector workers and instituting a policy that allowed employers to rescind time off, require overtime, and redeploy nurses anywhere they chose, demonstrated an absolute disregard for nurses and their work.[1] Yet Premier Ford continued to refer to us as "heroes" and make patronizing, sexist comments about how the Conservative Party loved "their nurses." Mr. Ford, I am not "your nurse," and despite what you may think, you do not own me.[2] The levee reference is used here metaphorically to describe how nurses have held healthcare systems together globally. As we are seeing now, this has not been sustainable. The pandemic highlighted the accumulated effect of devaluing and disregarding the nursing profession. Years of abuse from organizations, managers, patients, and now society have been too much to bear. When simply doing your job leads to verbal or physical abuse, a line is crossed for many nurses. Then add to this the decades-long healthcare budget cuts, cuts which nurses managed to deal with by always jumping in with solutions to manage with what we had.

Decisions are once again being made about nurses without having us at the table. Our initial education prepares us to be generalists, and from there we each go on to develop different specialties. You can't just pluck a critical care nurse from anywhere. Critical care nurses can take up to a year working in their setting, after completing a post-graduate certificate, to feel confident and competent. The Ford government believes we can shift homecare nurses into hospitals with no difficulty or rely on new graduates to fill the gap. These same new graduates may have never been in a hospital setting. I have heard frightening conversations regarding the use of new graduates and programs designed to educate and socialize nurses demonstrating an absolute lack of understanding of the knowledge and skill required to be a nurse.

The Canadian Institute for Health Information (CIHI) regularly publicizes information on health and human resources across Canada. In 2018, it was noted that Ontario had the worst nurse-to-patient population in all of Canada with only 669 nurses per 100,000 people, compared to 828 nurses to 100,000 in the rest of Canada.[3] For all of you Ontarians: there are not enough of us to care for all of you and that is a message that has failed to get out. Years and years of healthcare cuts borne on the back of nurses have led to our current realities. We have watched cyclical nursing shortages with no long-term planning despite some brilliant nursing researchers raising the alarm bells. These choices are political. Healthcare costs are too high, so let's cut nurses!

We know that our new graduates need at least two to five years to really solidify their knowledge and expertise, yet many leave areas such as medical and surgical units within the first two years of practice. There are lots of factors behind their decisions, including that we as members of the profession do not always treat our new graduates well. But by and large, these new nurses leave to take other positions, go back to graduate school, or become nurse practitioners. And while this is good, it is also a reflection of how our current systems and structures have been burning nurses out even before the pandemic hit. We are failing nurses and the nursing profession.

Nurses are the last line of defence; they are the canary in the coal mine. We are the ones there at 3:00 in the morning when all hell breaks loose. We are the ones who will take one look at you and, before you say a word, know what is going on. I can walk into a room and know without swabbing a wound what type of infection you have simply by the smell. I can pick up respiratory distress by looking at you and talking to you. Similarly, I can pick up emotional and psychological distress doing the same thing. I have spent hours on a shift trying to find someone to care for the pets of a patient admitted for emergency surgery so they could settle and focus on recovery. Where is that acknowledged? We are the calm in the storm. The ones who eyeball a patient walking through the door and immediately start setting up for the code we know is about to happen. In rural and remote areas, nurses are often the only healthcare provider, reaching physicians by phone, working at times with limited supplies, and innovating and making do.

I began my career in the HIV/AIDS pandemic of the late 1980s and 1990s and carry with me to this day the faces of the young men who died in my care. I was socialized as a new nurse during the era of the Mike Harris government, when I was told by Premier Harris that "a nurse is a nurse is a nurse" while comparing the work I did to that of a pastry chef. I watched as our healthcare system and my profession was decimated as Harris's Conservatives made drastic and dangerous changes. Harris believed that you could move nurses around from place to place as though they were widgets. This must be a conservative talking point because it has certainly been echoed by the Ford government.

Becoming a nurse was not my initial career plan, despite coming from a family of nurses, including aunts, cousins, and great-aunts, one of whom served in the Second World War with her brothers. I never regretted my decision, though, even during those difficult "Harris years," which effectively defined my career. That is until now.

Ironically, being around some amazing nurse leaders during the Harris era has influenced my own advocacy for and within my profession. As I reach the final stages of my career, I am even more determined to address these issues to make things better for my communities.

The cycle repeats: I am the mother of a new nurse who finds herself beginning her career in a pandemic with a premier and provincial government that show no understanding or valuing of the work of nurses in Ontario. I did not worry that I was going to die or be traumatized by my work; I can't say the same for my daughter.

For the last twenty plus years, I have taught nursing students. In 2020–1, most of my work was spent calming the fears of my students: fears about the virus and fears about going out into clinical environments unprepared. It was a tough line to walk, balancing the need to educate and prepare students, yet not fan their already significant fears. And now as I prepare yet again for another academic year in a pandemic, I am wondering: How the hell am I supposed to educate new nurses and get them excited to become a nurse while feeling like I am leading them to the slaughter?

To great fanfare, including a pronouncement from the Princess of Wales, Kate Middleton, the World Health Organization declared 2020 the "Year of the Nurse," a year to celebrate our profession at an international level.[4] Instead, it may have been the year the levee finally broke.

In considering where to go from here, I suggest we need to start by asking nurses what should be done. If one considers the history of nursing in Canada, it began in communities, with nurses seen as valued, knowledgeable providers making a difference in outcomes. There are so many contributions that nurses of all types could make to address this current healthcare crisis. In countries such as Britain, Ireland, Scotland, Australia, and New Zealand, the knowledge and skills of nurses are recognized and valued, with care delivery approaches that build upon that knowledge and skill. Nurses need to work in a setting that feels safe and supportive. There are numerous examples of team-based approaches in these countries, in which nurses are key partners, yet we are not provided with a seat at the table to discuss this.

The silence on display from Premier Ford and his cabinet regarding the nursing shortage is baffling. Worse, though, is the gaslighting: the comments regarding nurses, the premier and other party leaders disappearing for weeks at a time, not addressing pay rates, not addressing emergency room closures, and, worse, proposing actions that are based on how to "use nurses." We witness the lack of true political will to consider how to do things differently, within a publicly funded healthcare system, led by those doing the work. "Nurses Know" was a tagline of one of our nursing associations, yet it is so reflective of realities. Nurses do know; now we need decision-makers to listen to us.

It is time for decision-makers at all levels to see the value of nurses, including the public. Commentary that indicates we signed up for this, or that nurses already make too much money, continues to erode those working on the front lines. I was fortunate during my master's degree at the University of Toronto to be exposed to the brilliant work of Dr. Linda Lee O'Brien-Pallas who was working diligently to develop tools that would adequately measure and articulate the work of nurses. Specifically, she was working on a project to develop "nurse-sensitive outcomes," which would be attached to important measures such as patient length of stay and readmissions. These tools were developed in the early 2000s and have not yet been implemented.

Imagine how the system might look if we linked patient outcomes to the work of nurses, for instance, noting that a person who just had their hip replaced was discharged earlier than expected because of the care, assessment, and interventions applied by nurses. I suspect that would put an end to the short-sighted budgetary reactions of facilities that lay nurses off when their budgets are in the red.

Doug Ford has articulated, by his actions, or lack thereof, the Conservative government view of nurses in the province of Ontario. If there is truly interest in resolving this crisis, there needs to be a tremendous effort to heal the nursing profession.

KIM ENGLISH, RN, MN, EDD (C), is a professor at the Trent/ Fleming School of Nursing. She has expertise in nursing leadership and advocacy and rural and remote nursing practice.

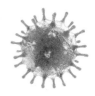

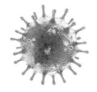

PART IV

NO SIMPLE FIXES

The final section of Breaking Canadians tells the story of the pandemic from the perspective of physicians, long-term care advocates, healthcare scholars and historians, and epidemiologists. These are some of the prominent Canadians who continue to speak out locally, provincially, federally, and internationally, to question our leaders' irresponsibility as they gaslight health experts and community advocates. They question the premise that we are "all in this together," and analyse how politicians and policymakers redefine "normalcy." They speak about their experiences of harassment, and the threats to their lives and livelihoods.

The book ends with a comparison of the politics and policies in previous pandemics. We cannot understand the present without examining the past and discerning our patterns, nor can we change our trajectory unless we commit to action. We must address global health disparities, and challenge the spread of disinformation, science illiteracy, and populism.

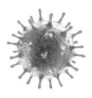

"We're All in This Together": COVID-19 and Principles of Environmental Justice

DR. JANE E. McARTHUR

We're all in this together. This phrase was an oft-heard one in the early weeks and months of the SARS-CoV-2 pandemic. It also happens to be the title of a song from *High School Musical*[1] and the one that my children loved, so the lyrics frequently rolled through my head and off my tongue as I reinforced why our lives had changed so significantly after the pandemic was declared.

I sang the words in response to my children's frustration – in the lingering weeks of online school, when they missed seeing their friends in person, and on video calls with family members – emphasizing that this was a just and ethical response to a global health crisis. In part, because my children and I had been active on issues of climate justice and environmental health, they already had an understanding of the value of cooperative action for shared well-being.

At the heart of the mantra *we're all in this together* is the notion of collective health and well-being, with the inference that limiting contacts, "social distancing," wearing masks, and reducing in-person activities was to everyone's benefit.[2] The message was an important public health signifier, and a call to action, even if it rang hollow for so many for whom COVID-19 was an amplifier of already existing inequities and exclusion.[3]

Underlying the message *we're all in this together* is also the idea of environmental justice. The US Environmental Protection Agency defines environmental justice as "the fair treatment and meaningful involvement of all people regardless of race, color, national origin, or income with respect to the development, implementation, and enforcement of environmental laws, regulations, and policies."[4]

Understanding what environmental justice is in theory and practice makes clear that the approach is about each of us and all of us. An exploration of how COVID-19 has been handled shines a light on the principles of environmental justice – including violations of the principles – and the injustices that pandemic impacts have produced.

As we continue to confront the SARS-CoV-2 pandemic, advocacy for virus and harm prevention in an environmental justice framework would shift the focus from the current personal risk assessment or "you do you"[5] approach to a truly "all in this together" attitude.

Principles of Environmental Justice

The seventeen Principles of Environmental Justice first outlined by the delegates to the First National People of Color Environmental Leadership Summit held in 1991 in Washington, DC, have served as a defining document in the movement for environmental justice.[6] Some of the key principles are particularly apt for understanding how the application of an environmental justice framework would have and still could change the shape of the COVID-19 pandemic and, in particular, the disproportionate health and other impacts experienced by some communities and people:

- Principle two "demands that public policy is based on mutual respect and justice for all peoples, free from any form of discrimination or bias."
- Principle five "affirms the fundamental right to political, economic, cultural and environmental self-determination of all peoples."
- Principle eight "affirms the right of all workers to a safe and healthy work environment without being forced to choose between an unsafe livelihood and unemployment. It also affirms the right of those who work at home to be free from environmental hazards."
- Principle nine "protects the right of victims of environmental injustice to receive full compensation and reparations for damages as well as quality health care."
- Principle ten "considers governmental acts of environmental injustice a violation of international law, the Universal Declaration on Human Rights, and the United Nations Convention on Genocide."
- Principle sixteen "calls for the education of present and future generations which emphasizes social and environmental issues, based on our experience and an appreciation of our diverse cultural perspectives."[7]

The violation of these principles can be illustrated in an examination of some of the phenomena that have occurred through the course of and the continued unfolding of the COVID-19 pandemic. And the value of understanding how to better apply the principles going forward can provide a framework for illness prevention, health promotion, and environmental justice for all.

While there is environmental justice work happening in Canada, more is needed in law, policy, and practice. The right to a healthy environment is now recognized under Canadian federal law with the June 13, 2023, passage of Bill S-5 to reform the Canadian Environmental Protection Act (CEPA),[8] which is consistent with the 2022 UN General Assembly declaration that a healthy environment is a human right.[9] And Bill C-226 when passed will be the first step in a national legal strategy to address environmental racism and environmental injustice in Canada, including the establishment of an Office of Environmental Justice.[10]

A concerted framework for environmental justice is necessary to address the climate crisis, toxic exposures, environmental racism, gaps in the protection of Indigenous Peoples, health inequalities and social determinants of health, and to prevent COVID-19. Integrating this human rights lens into decision-making and policy around COVID-19 would reinforce the environmental justice principles being applied to other environmental health issues.

Worker Health and Safety and COVID-19: Connecting the Dots on Injustice

The pandemic began just as I finished the analysis of the interviews for my doctoral research project with women workers at the Ambassador Bridge, which connects Windsor, Ontario, to Detroit, Michigan.[11] They suffered adverse health effects, particularly extremely high breast cancer rates, that scientific literature connects with environmental exposures.[12] I was researching and writing about the precautionary principle,[13] critiquing the responsibilization of women for their breast cancers,[14] exposing barriers in governance and disproportionate power relations that put women at risk,[15] and the problem of environmental injustice as it related to breast cancer incidence and survival.

In the midst of that, in the early spring of 2020, I began working with a team of researchers examining protections for healthcare workers when the science of airborne transmission of COVID-19 was already being documented in the scientific literature and being ignored by policymakers.[16]

The similarities between what women workers at the Ambassador Bridge told me about barriers to protection and what workers faced in the healthcare system were striking. I applied the principles and concepts from my breast cancer research to the unfolding of the pandemic, contributing to the public conversations about the precautionary principle,[17] collective responsibilities for health,[18] and the confusion created by the dichotomous approaches of personal responsibility and public health to environmental health risks.

It seemed straightforward to connect the dots between the challenges of controlling harmful exposures to toxic substances at work and in the environment and the issue of the denial of the airborne transmission of the novel coronavirus.[19] Seeing them as connected reinforced that not all exposures can be controlled through individual action and that exposures and outcomes are inequitably experienced. Improved policy and practices at levels outside the scope of personal control were and are necessary for the prevention of illness and to align with the principles of environmental justice.

Healthcare Workers

The example of healthcare workers is apt for understanding the application of environmental justice principles to COVID-19. For example, principle eight, which "affirms the right of all workers to a safe and healthy work environment without being forced to choose between an unsafe livelihood and unemployment," was and arguably still is being ignored in healthcare settings, including hospitals and long-term care facilities. An intersectional lens[20] also leads to the recognition that healthcare workers are often from marginalized communities, are underpaid, and face employment precarity, bringing into view principle two, which "demands that public policy is based on mutual respect and justice for all peoples, free from any form of discrimination or bias."

In the spring of 2020, as we were collecting and analysing healthcare worker testimonies of the conditions and protections in the face of COVID-19, the media were reporting that the pandemic was an unprecedented event. However, our research team argued that casting this crisis as exceptional narrowed the focus and omitted some critical elements of what workers were facing.

While the virus that causes COVID-19 was novel, the lack of preparedness and inadequate protection for healthcare workers was an old story. In many ways, it was an escalation of the ongoing failure of health and safety regulatory oversight and underscored chronic underfunding and increasing privatization in the healthcare sector. It was and is also an environmental justice problem.

In Canada, many healthcare workers are women, and many are recent immigrants or racialized and, in the early months, they represented a substantial proportion of COVID-19 cases. The politics and power relations in the workplace emerged as critical issues for these workers, which led to psychological distress and inadequate protection against an airborne virus, issues that added to inconsistencies in policy, government failings, and barriers to achieving needed changes. Healthcare workers described feeling powerless as individuals and at odds with their employers and governments.

We published our findings and later joined with researchers across the globe whose research had similar findings.[21] The healthcare workforces studied were predominantly women and significantly racialized. The workers included doctors, nurses, specialist technicians and professionals, aides, housekeeping, food service, and more. Their workplaces are hierarchical, and healthcare workers who spoke up for themselves or the people they care for reported that they faced threats, reprisals, and derision.

We collaborated on an international public statement,[22] which included seven calls to action to address infection, death, overwork, and stress of healthcare workers worldwide, starting with the assertion that governments must acknowledge that airborne particles transmit SARS-CoV-2, that they revise guidelines accordingly, and that they ensure accountability and strict regulatory enforcement. We finished with the demand that the final report of the SARS Commission of Canada be used as a roadmap, including its calls to respect the precautionary principle, involve the workforce in decision-making, and prepare well in advance of future pandemics.[23]

Dr. Michelle Ananda-Rajah, a physician in Melbourne, Australia, was one of our international collaborators. She powerfully asserted that "the WHO's denial of the airborne spread of this virus has given governments an excuse to deny [healthcare workers] appropriate protection across the world. It needs to be called out because this is not going to be the only pandemic we face in our lifetimes."[24] Healthcare standards leader Barry Hunt has reminded us that concentrations of viruses in hospital air are higher in less ventilated spaces and universal respirator use by healthcare workers, patients, and visitors would practically eliminate airborne transmission of all diseases in hospitals.[25]

Following the science of airborne transmission would better protect healthcare workers and patients.

The failure of governments to protect healthcare workers and the public they treat and serve is an act of environmental injustice and a violation of principle ten, which "considers governmental acts of environmental injustice a violation of international law, the Universal Declaration on Human Rights, and the United Nations Convention on Genocide."

Air Pollution

The connection between exposure to air pollution and COVID-19 also illustrates the problem of environmental injustice. In the first instance, environmental justice principle one is violated by the serious effects of air pollution on the health of the planet, compromising "the sacredness of Mother Earth, ecological unity and the interdependence of all species, and the right to be free from ecological destruction."

Human health is adversely affected by pollutants in the air.[26] Research suggests causal associations between air pollution exposure and a number of illnesses: reduction in healthy lung function, asthma, and other respiratory diseases; cardiovascular diseases; neurological disorders; pregnancy-related complications, including congenital abnormalities, infertility, and eclampsia; cancers, diabetes, obesity; dermatological diseases; and elevated mortality rates.

Air pollution and environmental inequality are also related. The health risks associated with air pollution are disproportionately experienced in communities with higher levels of pollution,[27] which are often also communities where racialized, Indigenous, and impoverished people live. Research has shown that air pollution increases COVID-19 infection, transmission, and the risk of COVID-19–related mortality.[28] This reality is a violation of principle five, which "affirms the fundamental right to political, economic, cultural and environmental self-determination of all peoples" because often the people exposed to air pollution and experiencing COVID-19 have little to no control over their environments and social factors.

The Canadian Association of Physicians for the Environment's (CAPE) report *Mobilizing Evidence: Activating Change on Traffic-Related Air Pollution (TRAP) Health Impacts*,[29] along with a study by Zander Venter and colleagues,[30] notes that substantial reductions in transportation-related air pollutants were realized during the pandemic's early months as a result of restrictions and lockdowns that targeted transportation and travel. This demonstrates society's capacity to implement effective public health and policy changes and the promise of working for policies and laws that can address environmental justice.

The intersections between exposure to air pollution, socio-economic factors, racialization, and severity of COVID-19 continue to be brought out in studies in Canada, the United States,[31] and other places across the globe. As ethicist Jon Parsons argues, "The current mass infection approach is an act of exclusion, first of all for what are called vulnerable people – disabled people, older adults, or anyone with compromised immune systems … Such exclusion is justified, either explicitly or implicitly, by assuming there are acceptable sacrifices of numbers of infections, hospitalization, long covid, and deaths. The idea is that it is okay that some are excluded or sacrificed so that others can 'live their life.'"[32]

Tolerating ongoing transmission of COVID-19 through the lack of public health policies that build on the knowledge of transmission and prevention tools perpetuates environmental injustices. Paired with the evidence that air pollution in already vulnerable communities – including those with higher racialized populations – exacerbates COVID-19 incidences and outcomes, these conditions produce situations where there are violations of multiple environmental principles, including principles two, five, and ten.

Social Factors Influence Health

The implication that individuals are responsible for or are to blame for health problems has been exposed for its deep flaws as we have watched COVID-19 kill residents and healthcare workers in long-term care facilities, infect healthcare workers, disproportionately impact racialized people, hit migrant farmworkers and precarious workers in service and retail, hospitalize children, and so much more. Personal responsibility is not a public health strategy.

Public health, as coined in the early nineteenth century,[33] is intended to distinguish the actions that governments and societies, as opposed to individuals, should take to protect people's health. COVID-19 – especially the denial that the virus is airborne and that there are disproportionate impacts on marginalized and vulnerabilized populations – has starkly illustrated what we have seen in environmental and occupational health struggles for decades: governance very much matters to health, and policies that fail to protect people are unjust.

As the examples of healthcare work and air pollution suggest, the COVID-19 crisis has made more visible and exacerbated links between racism, poverty, and health while providing opportunities to enact change for environmental justice.

Thinking about COVID-19 as an environmental justice problem begs us to recognize the nestedness of health – as is captured in the ecological view.[34] Ecological models "are concerned with the processes and conditions that govern the lifelong course of human development in the actual environments in which human beings live" and seek to account for the dynamic interplay between individual-level factors and social, political, and economic factors of the systems in the environment through the life course.[35]

The ecological model illustrates that health is not simply an outcome of behaviours and choices but that all our environments interact to produce risk or promote health. We can think about this model as social determinants of health or public health – which also inform the social justice elements inherent in health.

The omission of airborne science in messaging about COVID-19 and the corresponding inadequate protective and preventive action in our communities, public spaces, workplaces, and educational settings are environmental justice issues – and they are problems of governance, politics, and the complexity of our socio-ecological environments as they relate to health.

Focusing on preventing COVID-19 through individual choice and personal risk assessments ignores the nestedness of health. We don't all share equal access to the tools needed to prevent COVID-19, nor to the disproportionate exposures or inequitable conditions some populations face.

The ecological model shows that systemic changes and structural contributions such as policy, legislation, and practices in our work environments and communities are spaces where public health and prevention interventions are tools for social and environmental justice. This should include ventilation and filtration mandates, provision of respirators, testing, tracing and isolating, transparent data collection and sharing, and addressing conditions that make some people more susceptible to harm than others.

Moving Forward Together through an Environmental Justice Lens

The scientific evidence of airborne transmission of the virus that causes COVID-19 led to physician epidemiologist Dr. David Fisman's statement that "air is the new poop."[36] Just as clean water became a public health and political priority with the discovery of water-borne diseases such as cholera, typhoid, and more, COVID-19 begs us to take concerted action to clean the air indoors and outdoors for all environmental health hazards. Clean air – a healthy environment – is a right that should be afforded to all people, and one that the UN adopted in July 2022 when it passed its resolution declaring access to a clean, healthy, and sustainable environment a universal human right.[37]

With the scientific knowledge of the causes and conditions in our environments that lead to ill health, and disproportionate impacts on already vulnerabilized populations, plans for preventive action become possible, and so too does the realization of environmental justice. We have seen this reflected in the positive actions and advocacy by many who recognized the injustices the pandemic exacerbated.

Action and advocacy included outreach for a greater understanding of airborne transmission, increasing access to
vaccines for underserved communities, links made between
the disproportionate incidence of COVID-19 in racialized
and poor communities, accessibility of testing and rapid
antigen tests (RATs), social media campaigns outlining the
science of masks and respirators as well as ventilation and
filtration benefits, and programs for the distribution of free
N95 respirators – and much of this awareness-raising and
advocacy was undertaken by physicians and other healthcare providers who understood all too well the impacts on
people and the overburdened healthcare system.

As sociologist and professor in the Global Peace and
Social Justice Program at McMaster University, Dr. Ingrid
Waldron stated: "environmental policies are created by
members of the elite, mostly white people, who hold per-
ceptions about who matters and who does not matter."[38]
Building on Dr. Waldron's words, it's time for environmental justice policies – whether for airborne transmission of
COVID-19, environmental racism, exposures to toxins, or
climate change mitigation – that will prevent ill health and
uphold the right to a healthy environment for all. These policies must be created by those who work through the lens of
environmental justice.

Sadly, the *we're all in this together* sentiment has largely
been abandoned by public health messengers, the media,
and many people in general. But interrogating the idea provides a view to understanding how the pandemic has been
handled and how to move forward with a more protective
and preventive framework. This elucidation can put us on

track for a more just response to COVID-19 and other environmental health harms.

It is my hope that together we will advocate for policy decisions that would help us to fulfil the environmental justice principles, beginning with talking about and addressing how the pandemic response has been unjust. These conversations will be one way to live up to principle sixteen, which "calls for the education of present and future generations which emphasizes social and environmental issues, based on our experience and an appreciation of our diverse cultural perspectives."

JANE E. McARTHUR is the toxics program director with the Canadian Association of Physicians for the Environment (https://cape.ca/), a physician-led NGO that takes action to enable health for all by engaging with governments, running campaigns, conducting research, and drawing media attention to key issues to work effectively and build power together.

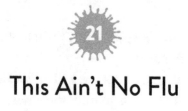

This Ain't No Flu

DR. STEVE FLINDALL

When I first heard reports of a novel coronavirus coming out of China, I remember scoffing to our chief of staff that this would probably turn out to be like a bad flu and everything would blow over in a couple of months, like it did with swine flu and avian flu. However, disastrous reports started to flow in from Italy and Iran, and I began to worry. Once very ill patients began flooding our emergency department, it dawned on me that this could be the pandemic that the medical community had worried was coming for decades and, possibly, the largest crisis of a generation.

The COVID-19 pandemic affected almost every facet of my life. Unlike many, I couldn't just stay home, learn a new hobby, and wait for restrictions to end so I could "get back to my life." Along with all acute care healthcare workers, I was tasked with fighting this unknown deadly virus that was sweeping the globe. I intentionally paid more attention to the media. I even opened a Twitter account for the first time, as I had been told that some of the most up-to-date and cutting-edge information about the novel coronavirus, as it was then called, was being shared on that platform. Stories about physicians, nurses, and respiratory therapists being infected and, in many cases, dying from this strange new virus abounded.

I was working in a large suburban community hospital in the Greater Toronto Area and, as cases began to come to our hospital, our emergency staff struggled with protocols that ranged from do we hold compressions on a patient with absent vital signs until they can be transported to an isolation room to whether we need an N95 mask while examining or even intubating patients suspected of being infected with COVID-19. A truly terrifying decision that faced us was if we needed to limit personal protective equipment (PPE) use and even recycle high-quality masks in the face of a possible shortage. Despite recommendations that had come out after the review of the original SARS outbreak that had affected Toronto area hospitals in 2003, the government had literally thrown stockpiles of PPE into refuse heaps without replenishing them. The very real fear that any of us might, on any given day, accidentally bring the virus home and infect our families loomed large.

Cases exponentially multiplied. Public health's ability to test suspected cases and even contact confirmed cases was outstripped. Again, the Ontario provincial government had myopically cut funding to public health in the very recent past, leaving us shorthanded in an area that was now desperately needed. Since no other physicians associated with our hospital volunteered, it fell to the Emergency Department (ED) to both run testing centres and follow-up on contact tracing for every case picked up at our hospital facilities. This added staffing pressures in the face of possible staff shortages due to illness.

Because no other group volunteered, the ED was again tasked with going to long-term care facilities and group homes to test residents in the centres that were experiencing outbreaks. With only a couple of exceptions, emergency physicians again stepped up to meet the challenge.

Guess who was tapped to run our mass vaccination centre? Then our Code Blue and Rapid Response Teams when our new facility was transformed into a COVID-19 receiving centre because hospitals were overwhelmed? Each time, our group responded with a positive "can-do" attitude.

After each shift, I had taken to showering and putting on fresh clothes before leaving the hospital to try to keep this mysterious virus with unknown properties of contagion from entering my house and infecting my family. No matter how exhausted I was, this seemed like a simple measure. Some healthcare workers were much more proactive: stories of workers sleeping and isolating in basements or even going so far as to rent other properties or house trailers that they parked in their driveways. I will not fault anyone for taking whatever precautions they felt necessary at the time. How would any of us have felt if we brought the virus into our households and one of our family members was infected and died? It was not an unsubstantiated fear. I personally resuscitated the spouse of a healthcare worker that came to us after suffering a cardiac arrest as the result of a COVID-19 infection they contracted through the worker. We were successful in the ED but, ultimately, the patient had such significant neurologic injury that life support was withdrawn a few days later.

Since the birth of our first child, my wife and I had intended to draw up our wills. That was about fifteen years prior to the onset of the COVID-19 pandemic. As events and stories like the one above circulated, I told my wife we had to get our affairs in order. We were lucky enough to find an estate lawyer who helped us over the phone and internet. On a chilly spring morning, we met with this very generous woman in her garage to sign our last wills and testaments. It was not the highlight of my year, but it did feel like quite a relief to get it done.

The cases of COVID-19 kept coming and, with them, the stress. This was all on top of the baseline stress that we usually experience in the ED. Eventually, it started to become too much for some. I came to work one day, and a nurse told me that one of our excellent nurses had just applied for a transfer. I had worked with this man for more than half a decade and he was an excellent, proficient, and dedicated veteran nurse. He had all the qualities you want in a member of your team. It wasn't a COVID-19 case that was the final straw. It was a two-year-old that came in dead after a trauma that we could not save. The unrelenting stress of the pandemic had left him unable to cope with that loss. It was the first time I saw a good nurse leave during the pandemic, but it was certainly not the last. All the factors contributing to nurse attrition are described in discussions elsewhere in painful detail but the stress of COVID-19 was the final straw for many veteran nurses.

As cases continued to mount throughout 2020, it seemed odd to me that many of our public health and political leaders seemed to be signalling that things in hospitals were improving. Indeed, new cases were slowing but the number of ill patients coming to the ED had not slowed at all. Importantly, the number of patients in our intensive care unit (ICU) continued to climb. What had not been anticipated prior to the onset of COVID-19 was just how long patients that required intensive care would continue to require those services. Some patients needed extraordinary measures such as dialysis or extracorporeal circulatory support (a process where patients are essentially put on a cardiac bypass machine to keep their blood oxygenated because their heart and/or lungs are unable to do so). An ICU's occupancy was a key indicator for whether a hospital would become overwhelmed. Both politicians and medical professionals recognized the likely pattern that was to unfold: cases followed by hospitalized patients followed by lengthy ICU occupancy followed by deaths. Even though cases dropped, as the politicians claimed, the ICUs remained full, people died, and hospitals were overwhelmed.

To my mind, this is where the solidified effort in trying to control COVID-19 started to collapse, and public opinion splintered. Politicians began talking about the negative impact public health measures were having on the economy and media outlets started featuring stories about struggling small business owners. I knew Ontarians were in trouble from a public health standpoint when I saw our premier, Doug Ford, at a press conference around this time. Ford has a habit of speaking with an odd sing-song cadence when he is delivering prepared speeches. In the earliest days of the pandemic, that sing-song quality was gone, and he seemed to be speaking out of genuine concern and with true human emotion. By December 2020, the sing-song was back in Doug Ford's voice: "My friends," he said, and I knew a corner had been turned and Ford was back to being more politician than human.

At this press conference, Ford announced that different public health authorities would be allowed, at the discretion of the local medical officer of health (MOH), to reopen amenities in their region. My MOH chose to open large shopping centres. I was stunned. After a particularly busy evening in the ED, I decided to tweet about how busy our ED was, and how stressed and overwhelmed our nursing staff was. This tweet attracted a lot of attention. I was asked to give several interviews for radio and newspaper outlets. This, in turn, led to some television news outlet interviews. To my relief, the hospital I was working for, although not wild about the attention I was receiving, was not telling me to be quiet. In fact, several high-placed individuals in the organization thanked me for speaking out and said they wished they could be as candid as I was being.

Then came the inevitable backlash. A close colleague put out a counter tweet implying I was exaggerating the matter. People who had lost income and businesses targeted me. I didn't blame them. I understood they were suffering. What truly baffled me were the people in and around healthcare who should have known better and who were minimizing what I and many other physicians and related healthcare professionals were trying to make the public aware of.

Regulatory bodies seemed reluctant to act against physicians who were blatantly contradicting medical knowledge and public health policy. Some physicians were clearly marketing their own personal brand to monetize the pandemic. Still, little was done to curb disinformation.

Then came a miracle: vaccines had cleared clinical trials and were showing tremendous results. I was asked during an interview at the time what I thought of the vaccines. My response, and I still maintain this opinion, was that it was the greatest scientific achievement of the last fifty years. In less than a year we had gone from a mysterious illness causing the deaths of thousands in China to a clinically validated vaccine that showed greater than 95 per cent efficacy at preventing serious illness and death. Outstanding! We were saved! Of course, it didn't quite play out that way.

Every health professional I knew jumped at the chance to get a dose of the vaccine. My colleagues and I received some of the first doses given in the province. We rapidly set up a mass vaccination clinic. People were elated. However, after a few months, a sense of discord started to emerge. Initially, people were having trouble accessing the vaccine. Not much later, a reluctance of some individuals to become vaccinated appeared. The government then started, as it had historically with other diseases like mumps, tuberculosis, polio, and smallpox, to implement mandates requiring individuals in certain sectors to be vaccinated. Despite vaccine mandates being a part of societal norms for decades, many were outraged by these "new" rules.

As the debate raged on, COVID-19 cases kept mounting. Many hospitals became overwhelmed with cases and no

longer had the ICU capacity to care for their own populations. ICU patients were transferred throughout the province from hospitals with no ICU space to those with some
capacity. Our hospital was to open a second site with an
entirely new Emergency Department, outpatient services,
and inpatient units. Instead, it was designated a COVID-19
relief centre. We used our inpatient facilities, especially the
ICU, to take patients from around the province. Our internal
medicine colleagues were maxed out and unable to provide
twenty-four-hour coverage for critical care services at the
new site. Many of our emergency physicians volunteered to
help by providing back-up care, especially overnight. While
we had the new facility, we were very low on staff and medical equipment.

I remember one night having a COVID-19 patient decom-
pensating and becoming increasingly hypoxic. When I requested a high-flow oxygen unit, I was told we had none. I
was also told that if I were to put her fully on a ventilator,
we had no more ICU space, and she would have to be transferred across the province to one of the only ICU beds left
in Ontario. Fortunately, we were able to manage by having the patient lie with her most affected side down so that
her good lung could keep oxygenating to its optimum. This
kept her stable overnight, long enough to free up a high-
flow unit for her. That was a tense night.

In the spring of 2022, case counts, inpatient cases, and
ICU cases dropped to the point where we could open the
new site as a full hospital. Despite having some of the most
affected demographics of the pandemic, we have one of the
highest rates of unvaccinated individuals in our catchment

area. Over the last year and a half, almost every single patient complaint I have received has been related to patients feeling that I didn't support them in their decision to remain unvaccinated. But how could I? I tried each time to explore their reasoning and explain why I thought they should get the vaccine. Apart from young women who had become fearful through the propagation of the lie that the vaccine would reduce their chance of having a viable pregnancy, every anti-vaxx patient I had would disavow science and spout some internet-derived rhetoric. There was no way I could possibly support their position. It was akin to asking a vegetarian to work in a steak house and smile while doing it.

Shockingly, the Ontario government and Public Health Ontario did not strongly push for vaccinations. They declined to make school vaccinations mandatory. The public education component for vaccines dropped to almost zero. It was so bad that many individuals who would qualify for boosters, or initial doses in the case of younger children, did not even realize they were eligible. The chief medical officer of health (CMOH) even went so far as to point out a rare, benign side effect of the vaccine, myocarditis, as a reason for people to choose to NOT be vaccinated. Mask mandates were dropped across the province. Hospitals were forced to implement and enforce their own mask mandates. Businesses that would have gladly supported ongoing masking were bullied and intimidated into dropping it as they had no support from public health authorities. The CMOH himself was then spotted at a public gathering without a mask on after advising masking under such circumstances.

This, of course, undermined his public messaging. Calls for complete independence for the position of the CMOH from political influence have thus far not been met with any enthusiasm from the government.

On top of official complaints, I continued to receive threats and insults over the internet. People who were not my patients went on Rate-Your-MD and gave me one-star ratings. Some were even humorous in their content. One person suggested that I give up medicine and start selling oral sexual favours near the largest train station in the country.

Airing grievances online was one matter, but having anti-vaxx encounters that were aggressive was quite another. One fellow who had clearly been at the Ottawa Freedom Convoy protests came in with symptoms of COVID-19. When I went to swab him, he slapped my hand away. The spouse of another patient who came in with COVID-19 and was in rough shape threatened to kill me if their partner died. The spouse felt that COVID-19 was a hoax. If their partner died, I was to blame for not prescribing antibiotics. The parent of an infant with a viral illness called me a fraud because I wanted to test the child for COVID-19.

Despite taking on the risk of treating an unknown deadly pathogen, then doing our best to educate and protect the public, healthcare workers are now too often seen as killjoys that are "living in fear" and trying to keep the rest of the populace from exiting the pandemic.

I've not lost a lot during the pandemic. I didn't lose my business, and no one close to me died of COVID-19. What I have lost is something more essential, though. I've lost my belief in a coherent society that will make small sacrifices to keep the vulnerable among us safe. I don't know if I'll ever get that belief in my fellow human beings back.

STEVE FLINDALL, MD, CCFP (EM), is an emergency physician who practises in York Region, Ontario, in high-volume community hospitals.

The Doctor as Advocate

DR. JOE VIPOND

But nothing worth having comes without some kind of fight,
Got to kick at the darkness 'till it bleeds daylight.
> – Bruce Cockburn, "Lovers in a Dangerous Time"

The *Merriam-Webster Dictionary*'s definition of advocacy is "the act or process of supporting a cause or proposal."[1] A simpler way of viewing the word is as an individual or organization trying to change the future. Imagine the future being a road, extending forward. Every policy or idea has a set course for the direction it is taking, which is generally to follow the status quo (a straight road). When one intervenes to change that course – through meetings, media, one-on-one conversations – it is an effort to change the course of action (bending the road).

A particular advocate is rarely alone in trying to influence action, or to change the direction of the road. There are generally advocates working to shift the path on all sides. The natural course is the status quo, and often the most powerful and resourced entities are working to protect this course. Typically, they have been enriched or have benefited from this course and are fearful of any variation, so have the most at stake in any change – although history often shows that the magnitude of the effect is often not as severe as feared, and sometimes even beneficial. Examples include the impact of pedestrian-only access to Times Square in New York City or the cost of compliance on acid rain regulations. Sometimes those in opposition will suddenly try to shift the curve in the opposite direction, causing a whiplash-like re-action. The summation of all the various forces acting on the direction of the road – advocacy, public sentiment, science, and governmental values – will determine its final course, and that of history.

For physicians like myself, advocacy can take place at three levels: the individual (advocating for a patient's path through the healthcare system); the institutional (our hospital needs to do better at paper recycling); and the systemic/political (requesting a coal phase out to decrease air pollution and greenhouse gas emissions). Advocacy is supposed to be a core competency for all physicians along with other roles such as scholar, expert, and leader. Yet of all the competencies, advocacy gets the least attention and fewest resources during our training and beyond.

The COVID-19 pandemic has seen an incredible burst of systemic advocates come on the scene from all directions: from anti-mask to anti-vaxx, all the way through to Zero COVID. As a physician and active citizen, I felt it was necessary to speak up, organize, and attempt to save lives, first in supporting mask use, then mandates, then opposing the rapid opening up of society as we entered the nadir of waves. It was an awkward position to be in as a non-academic clinical emergency physician, to be actively pushing those in public health to do more, faster, especially when they seemed far more influenced by economic and political concerns rather than by the health and science.

There were so many policy decisions that excluded scientific evidence. I found it overwhelming. In which direction should I focus my advocacy?

The first step was to gather allies. And there were many. In early May 2020, we assembled to form Masks4Canada, a grassroots group of healthcare workers, academics, and other professionals collaborating to advocate for evidence-based and equitable public-health measures during the COVID-19 pandemic.

A short but non-exhaustive list of topics that Masks4Canada and I have engaged in include:

- Mask use for PPE and source control
- Mask mandates
- Acknowledgment and mitigation of airborne transmission
- Respirator use by the public and in healthcare settings
- Importance of schools in community transmission
- Limiting infections among children
- Addressing transmission in racialized and lower socio-economic status groups

- Arguing for transparency on healthcare and public health data
- Rapid Antigen Test access for the public
- Vaccines for children
- Boosters for everyone
- Impossibility of a vaccine-only endgame strategy
- The existence of long COVID and its importance to our society
- Consideration of a Zero-COVID strategy
- National approach to policy over the fractured provincial/municipal approach (such as different definitions of "mask mandate" across the country)
- Privileging of ableism[2] and the impact of mitigation removal on the susceptible

Four Principles of Advocacy

The four most prominent principles that drove my advocacy and that of many of my colleagues were the precautionary principle; the role of asymptomatic COVID-19; the importance of long COVID; and airborne transmission.

Not one of these principles is currently reflected in public policy, even after more than three full years of disease.

The Precautionary Principle

Both the precautionary principle and airborne transmission mitigation feature prominently in the 2003 Ontario

SARS-CoV-1 report,[3] which breaks down the lessons from the original coronavirus outbreak. The precautionary principle is an overriding principle that if you have incomplete information about a situation, and there are severe consequences to following one path, always choose the path of the least amount of harm even if it means expenditure of resources or an impact on the economy. In environmental terms, it is often applied to the introduction of new chemicals: if there is the possibility of high-impact toxicity, best not to move ahead on approval before more is known on the topic. In the pandemic, it was best applied to the introduction of non-pharmacology interventions (or protections), such as masks or airborne mitigation.

Early on there was a strong resistance to the use of masks, the argument being that there was not enough scientific evidence to support their use by the public. But, applying the precautionary principle, it was clear that the risk of masking was far outweighed by the benefits of preventing viral transmission. There is now almost universal consensus that simple masks had an important role in preventing overwhelming transmission. But it is also clear that their use has been politicized to cause substantial polarization in society. It has also become clear that with the increased transmissibility of newer variants, simple masks are no longer adequate to prevent transmission and respirator-style masks are required.

The precautionary principle also would have been important to apply to mitigation in schools, the "let it rip" strategy of the Omicron outbreak, and many other aspects of the pandemic.

Asymptomatic COVID-19

Reports of asymptomatic transmission of the virus filtered out of Wuhan early in the pandemic and became evident with the *Diamond Princess* cruise ship outbreak. But curiously, the scientific community was slow to recognize this as a key element in the pandemic. Indeed, it was precisely the asymptomatic component that made this pandemic so very different from the 2003 SARS outbreak. In 2003, patients did not become infectious until symptoms appeared, therefore it was easier to contain: quarantine all sick people and their contacts. But with the new pandemic, the infectious walked among us, invisibly.

To be clear, there are three types of asymptomatic people: the true asymptomatic (those who never have symptoms), the pauci-symptomatic (those with very mild symptoms: Is that a sore throat or is it just a little sensitive today? I sneezed once, is that a symptom?), and the pre-symptomatic transmitters (those who will develop symptoms in a day or two but are currently breathing out the virus without symptoms). From a scientific perspective, there may be utility in differentiating the three, but from a policy perspective, there is one critical issue: you can't develop policies that focus on symptoms, like screening forms or temperature checks. People in all spaces need to be treated as potentially infectious, including yourself. This speaks to the need for mask mandates when viral levels are high. Everyone needs to wear a mask not only as personal protective equipment (PPE), but as source control, because any one of us in a space might be exhaling plumes of airborne virus.

Long COVID

Like so many aspects of the pandemic, long COVID was slow to be recognized by the scientific community despite many case reports being discussed early in the pandemic in the media and on social media. Just as with pre-pandemic chronic fatigue syndrome (myalgic encephalitis) and fibromyalgia, sufferers were told it was all in their heads and often labelled as having psychiatric disorders. It was only through constant advocacy by patients themselves that long COVID began to be treated as a true medical entity unto itself.

Long COVID isn't easy to pigeonhole, given there are over 200 symptoms affiliated with the moniker, but the result is the same: disability. With 10 to 50 per cent (depending on which paper you read) of unvaccinated people who become infected having some of the symptoms (perhaps halve this risk for the fully vaccinated), and a narrative that all of us are going to be infected eventually (now transitioning to "we're going to be infected multiple times, every year"), we cannot ignore the societal impacts of long COVID.

At an individual level, getting long COVID can be devastating, and there are innumerable stories online of the impact on people's lives, including divorce and even suicide. But at a societal level, it can be equally devastating, with reports of up to 50 per cent of those with long COVID being unable to work in their original jobs. Major banking institutions are now identifying long COVID as a key reason for the staffing crisis afflicting almost all industries, in almost all corners of the world, all at once. And we have yet to even begin the discussion of the financial issues and healthcare costs that go along with supporting this tsunami of individuals with disabilities.

Airborne Transmission

The airborne transmission discussion has been a difficult one and is still playing out.

Although there exists strong consensus among engineers, occupational hygienists, and policymakers – the World Health Organization,[4] Centers for Disease Control and Prevention,[5] Public Health Agency of Canada,[6] US Environmental Protection Agency,[7] ASHRAE,[8] and most recently the White House[9] – that airborne mitigation will be one of the most important next steps in limiting spread, through ventilation, filtration, and respiratory masks, we still lack the push needed to explain this to the public, and we still do not have any strong policy support being given to organizations and institutions to implement these measures. Every time I see hand sanitizer at the entrance to a store but no mask encouragement, or an institution that celebrates its regular deep cleaning, I am reminded of our failure as a society to truly attempt to mitigate transmission.

Costs of Advocacy

From the very beginning of the pandemic, I felt the need to step forward and push for better policy. It began with being confused by the recommendations from high-level public health and infectious disease physicians to not wear a mask to protect oneself and others. This flew in the face of common sense and what we were quickly learning about the behaviour of the virus in those countries earliest affected. My advocacy included writing op-eds, doing media, collecting scientific evidence, sharing on social media, gathering organizational and individual support, creating engaging and enlightening events, co-founding Masks4Canada, and meeting with politicians and policymakers.

My advocacy efforts have not been without risk to myself. From the right wing, there have been recurrent efforts to undermine my standing in society, from painting me as a political shill (I'm still waiting for my purported cheques from the NDP) to accusing me of hypocrisy when my online behaviour doesn't meet a particular standard that they have preset for me. There have been protests outside my house and hate graffiti on the sidewalk leading to my door. These attacks are generally more nuisance than anything, and the negative feedback is easily discounted as nonsense.

More worrisome are the attacks from institutions and leadership – to have my employment threatened for drawing attention to poor decisions. And I am not alone. I have heard of multiple colleagues threatened with similar actions. Predominant among the concerns is "undermining public health messaging." Most of these complaints are still in the process of being resolved. One would hope, in a democracy with freedom of speech, that there is room in a society for critical thought and analysis, especially during a pandemic where so many important truths have been recurrently ignored by leaders.

When your advocacy is successful, the rewards are great. You get to help change history and improve society. Aside from this inner reward, there is not a lot of incentive to do advocacy. It is not respected by educational institutions, who value research well above advocacy, it can damage relationships at work and in society, and it is generally not compensated financially. And because of a lack of training, most physicians do not feel competent in the specialized skills, such as communicating with the media, that are required of successful advocates. Perhaps this explains why, despite the large number of physicians in Canada, only a handful of them have stepped up to fill this role during this recent medical crisis.

All of this needs to change if we want a society where physicians successfully play a role in shaping policy. First, we must train budding physicians in the skills required: not only in critical thinking, so that the policies they advocate for are scientifically based, but also in media training, writing skills, and meeting management. Second, we need to pay more than lip service to advocacy as a key role for physicians and elevate this role in society. Finally, we need to protect advocates from vexatious complaints meant to silence these important voices.

Despite everyone's best hopes, with humans' inability (so far) to create sterilizing immunity, and rapid evolution of new immune evasive variants, the pandemic is not petering out. There will be new pandemics (likely driven by airborne transmission) and recurrent health crises, not to mention the ongoing and existential climate crisis and rising autocracy around the world. Physician advocate voices will be key to shaping policy going forward, and how we support them now will define how safe others will feel in stepping up when the need arises again. And again. And again. We need them because we need a better world, and they will help create the path to our desired future.

This chapter was written in May 2022, when Omicron had been circulating for six months.

DR. JOE VIPOND is an emergency physician who practises in Calgary, Alberta, the past-president of the Canadian Association of Physicians for the Environment, the co-founder of Masks4Canada and the Calgary Climate Hub, and a member of the John Snow Project.

Disability Rights and Advocacy

DR. CHRISTOPHER LEIGHTON

November 2022.

Post-Traumatic Flashbacks

In early March 2020, I knew what was about to befall Ontarians. I am a radiation oncologist who initially trained in Toronto at the height of the HIV/AIDS epidemic. As the COVID-19 pandemic began, I was flooded with horrible memories from the start of my career. Later, I was surprised to learn that this was not an uncommon response among healthcare workers.

Flashback to my first month as an internal medicine intern at the now-closed Wellesley Hospital's ICU. That year was a brutal education in treating immunocompromised people. Young men in their twenties and thirties with advanced-stage AIDS were being admitted, and then dying in front of me, sometimes two or three a shift. I was barely twenty-five years old, having been accepted to medical school after just two years of university.

I recall a high school teacher being admitted with advanced PCP (Pneumocystis carini pneumonia), for which there were no truly effective treatments at the time, especially for individuals with low lymphocyte counts. He was in his early thirties, conscious but on a ventilator. He was not responding to intravenous "Double Strength Septra," or inhaled pentamidine, our only therapeutic options at the time. We obtained a do-not-resuscitate (DNR) order. He signed papers. He had one family member/friend present; many had no one. He was sedated, his breathing tube was removed, and then he died. An hour later, another HIV patient took his bed. Also with PCP. The inpatient wards were full of young men dying from other HIV-related maladies. It was a nightmare. I am not sure I had ever truly processed my experiences. It's also a common coping mechanism for healthcare providers: We believe we are not vulnerable to our patients' illnesses, especially early in our careers.

I didn't appreciate post-traumatic stress disorder (PTSD) until COVID-19 hit. I couldn't sleep. I had anxiety and vivid flashbacks of individual patients that I hadn't recalled for twenty-five years. My mood became depressed. I became active on social media, Twitter largely, and read copious amounts about the emerging pandemic. I began to consider how my own world might change. I had studied epidemiology and biostatistics, but infectious disease epidemiology and public health were not areas to which I had exposure.

I soon learned that my personal risk of complications from infection might be high.

Physician Becomes Patient

I developed a strange viral illness just six months into my first staff position as a radiation oncologist at the age of twenty-nine. After a few weeks of flu-like symptoms, I awoke one morning feeling terribly unwell with paralysis of my left leg. I was admitted to hospital and initially diagnosed with a post-viral spinal cord inflammation. Years later, I was retrospectively diagnosed with inflammation of my brain and brain stem. In hospital, I had delirium for four days, improved, and was discharged ten days later, walking with a cane.

I recovered with rehabilitation and returned to my practice a few months later. Thirteen months later, I had a severe relapse that left me with a permanent disability and constant nerve pain in my face, torso, and extremities. My career was limited to half days thereafter. By 2008, I had developed frequent respiratory infections, and was diagnosed with an immunoglobulin deficiency. I was an immunocompromised person with an unknown neuroimmune disorder.

Self-Advocacy

It was an enormous challenge to work as a physician with a disability. It provided a thorough and unwanted look at the world through the eyes of a working disabled person. It was ugly. Even as a physician, several colleagues treated me as if I was carrying on with "back pain." I was verbally harassed by one physician colleague. Our cancer centre CEO related to me his "own" experience with the same extremely rare condition, and that he just bucked up and worked through the pain. (With only one in a million annual incidences, the odds were astronomically high that we, in fact, did not share the same condition.) Physicians are not necessarily the most compassionate to their own kin, especially if they fear the call schedule or their workload may be impacted. Compounding this early experience was the wide sharing of my medical record among non-physician colleagues. My imaging reports were available for all to read, and many did (before digital information was protected). It was widely assumed that I had multiple sclerosis. I did not.

I had to relocate cities twice to maintain my clinical career in oncology, reinvented myself with a focus on complex pain management and palliative care, and thereafter, transitioned my focus towards undergraduate medical education. Resistance to providing disability accommodations was not uncommon. Though my situation was generally accepted by my colleagues, I had several unpleasant experiences, most notably being denied promotion to associate professor in the Department of Oncology after the recommendation of the Promotions and Tenure Committee. It was a most unusual, if not unprecedented, occurrence in the history of our department.

I practised as a radiation oncologist for thirteen years; I worked twelve of those with an unpredictable disability and only did so with the help of skilled lawyers and the

protections provided by the Ontario Human Rights Code
(OHRC). I was constantly immersed in human rights law,
learning about the OHCR, tribunal complaints, and attempting to have workplace accommodations introduced.

Ableist Policies and Politics

Many disabled Canadians live in poverty without private
or group disability insurance. Few can afford attorneys.
The average experience is unemployment. This knowledge
inspired me to speak for the impoverished and voiceless
struck with a disability, especially as the pandemic took
hold in Ontario.

The pandemic raised the significant issue of poverty
amongst our severely disabled. One in four disabled Canadians live in poverty. Provincial support programs are
inadequate and relegate individuals to abject poverty, well
below Canada's poverty line by this author's review. Our
Ontario government had not provided these individuals
additional benefits, inflation adjustments, or even free N95
masks. They have been hit especially hard by COVID-19.

I wrote several letters to Prime Minister Trudeau and
Minister Carla Qualtrough urging them to pass the Canadian Disability Benefit Act, which would provide disabled
Canadians a benefit similar to the Guaranteed Income Supplement, thus putting them at par with income received by
low-income seniors.

I found myself advocating for better public health measures. We teach the "Heath Advocate" as a fundamental

competency of a physician. Like hundreds of other Ontario physicians, I felt that responsibility weigh on me, especially as an educator, a physician, and a vulnerable person.

I wrote letters to the minister of health and to public health officials, spoke to the media, and was interviewed by CBC television in August 2020. I petitioned local school boards to limit class sizes and improve ventilation after Dr. David Fisman, professor of public health at the University of Toronto, and Dr. Lindsey Marr, professor of engineering at Virginia Tech, had clearly made the convincing case that airborne spread contributed to SARS-CoV-2 transmission.

Later, my advocacy focused on the gross ableism apparent in the roll out of vaccinations in Canada. Initially, age was the only factor used as a determinant for vaccine eligibility. The evidence was apparent that other high-risk groups existed, especially those with Down's syndrome and organ transplant recipients. The United Kingdom and Israel included all individuals with significant comorbidities at the beginning of their vaccine campaigns. Canada did not. I petitioned our federal government, the National Advisory Committee on Immunization (NACI), and later, the Ontario Vaccination Task Force to consider other vulnerable risk groups. In March, I followed up with letters recommending the prioritization of vaccine delivery by risk groups (severe, moderate, and lower risk). I made suggestions to the Windsor-Essex medical officer of health, Dr. W. Ahmed, on how to approach prioritization in our area. I believe these latter suggestions were largely adopted.

I became especially concerned for those individuals vulnerable to COVID-19 infection in June 2022, after the

Ontario government removed all masking requirements in public buildings. In August 2022, practically all public health measures were withdrawn, ending masking in schools and removing isolation requirements while infectious, provided that symptoms were improving and any fever had resolved. At this time children ages five to eleven were largely unvaccinated, with 67 per cent lacking two mRNA vaccine doses. Many physicians were worried about a massive wave of illness after the return to school. The dissolution of the Ontario COVID-19 Advisory Science Table was alarming. Its scientific director, Dr. Fahad Razak, recommended masking for students in the fall in stark opposition to recommendations of the Ontario chief medical officer of health. I mobilized a group of public health experts and epidemiologists, a legal scholar, and those with careers in healthcare, law, and education. I sought advice, on or off the record, and in a few weeks had authored a collaborative twenty-six-page brief for the chief commissioner of the Ontario Human Rights Commission, which was signed by forty-seven physicians, nurses, scientists, and educators. We had requested an urgent section 31 inquiry (Ontario Human Rights Code, RSO 1990, c H.19, Section 31) into the decisions by the Ontario government to lift nearly all COVID-19 public health measures and suggested such an action that would increase the health risks to OHRC-protected, COVID-19–vulnerable Ontarians was contrary to the OHRC. We quoted sections of the Education Act and the Health Protection and Promotion Act that the government appeared to have violated and described government actions that appeared at odds with the

COVID-19 recovery planning policy of the Ontario Human Rights Commission.

Our petition was denied by the chief commissioner on 4 November 2022. The Honourable Patricia DeGuire stated: "The decision to begin an inquiry under section 31 of the Code is based on several factors as set out in the OHRC's Litigation and Inquiry Strategy criteria. The OHRC has concluded that it is not appropriate to undertake an inquiry into this matter. The Code provides various other tools that the OHRC may use, including policy statements."

I made a subsequent request for a specific accommodation policy that defined OHRC-protected individuals with respect to COVID-19, one which outlined the basic tenets for accommodation. Such a policy would make it easier for COVID-19 vulnerable Ontarians to request accommodations at school or in the workplace, and included four elements: ventilation, air filtration (HEPA), group masking (as in classrooms), and isolating while contagious. This request was also denied.

In October 2022, I filed a Freedom of Information request to the chief medical officer of health, Dr. Kieran Moore. I had requested all scientific information used by his office to make the decision to remove COVID-19 isolation requirements (twenty-four hours following resolution of fever) and all the evidence that he had relied upon that demonstrated one-way masking does not increase the risks to vulnerable persons. It was my position that if risks to the vulnerable were increased by this policy change, then it was his duty to publicly declare that risk. After two sixty-day extensions, a reply is now imminent, though significant redactions are expected.[1]

The fall of 2022 saw the worst paediatric critical care crisis in Ontario and across Canada. Severe RSV (respiratory syncytial virus) infections, influenza, and COVID-19 brought previously healthy children into children's hospitals everywhere. Large teaching hospitals in Ottawa and Toronto had to quickly expand critical care beds. Why? It's believed by many infectious disease specialists and immunologists that repeated COVID-19 infections among unvaccinated children caused immune dysregulation, contributing to more severe common infections. Reduced exposure to circulating viruses could explain more frequent infections but not for the severity observed. In fact, RSV prevalence in Ontario was no greater than in prior years. The phenomenon was seen with group A streptococcus also. Regrettably, 2022 was the deadliest year of the pandemic for adults and children in Canada. At the end of 2022, it remained the third leading cause of death.

Advocacy has never been more important. Ontario physicians were central to moulding the government response to the pandemic. Prioritization was made for at-risk groups, and the vulnerable were vaccinated (including myself in April 2020). Advocacy also helped me to cope with my own risk and self-imposed isolation. The public health failures were most troubling, and I wonder if we could have done anything else to lessen suffering.

We have the knowledge and ability to make all workplaces, schools, public transportation, and restaurants far safer with simple changes: improved ventilation and HEPA filtration. New accredited building standards would be akin to an invisible mask. It's an innovation that would place Canada in an advantageous position before the next pandemic. COVID-19 isn't leaving us anytime soon and the threats of long COVID will linger for years to come, not to mention the ongoing threat to the immunocompromised. Every Canadian can request that their elected officials adopt such recommendations.

Advocacy Matters

Our healthcare system has always relied on strong advocates. Physicians must speak for the vulnerable. We do so in our daily clinical practices. For example, in my brain tumour practice, I was accustomed to rushing my patients' MRI appointments, having them reprioritized if necessary, and then reviewing the scan with the radiologist in person, before it was reported. There are times when speed matters. It is a lesson that was and is difficult for our governments to learn.

As I learned of the disparate roll out of the vaccine in early in 2021, leaving out those who were disabled or with congenital syndromes, I was frankly enraged. Ableism is entrenched within our society. NACI – the National Advisory Committee on Immunization – had initially ignored the risks of COVID-19 to people with disabilities, and the Ontario provincial government vaccine roll out was going to follow suit. Advocacy made a difference. I hope I have raised awareness about the vulnerable who have been especially impacted by this pandemic.

One does not need to experience any of my life events to be an effective advocate, thank goodness. However, we do need to care for one another, and speak for the voiceless. I plan to continue to do so.

CHRISTOPHER LEIGHTON, MD, FRCPC, is a radiation oncologist on long-term disability. He is also adjunct professor of oncology at the Schulich School of Medicine and Dentistry, University of Western Ontario.

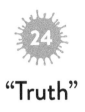

"Truth"

DR. IMOGEN COE

Vaccines save lives.

Regardless of your age or background, being scientifically literate is empowering.

These simple statements are fundamental truths and, before the pandemic, I would have assumed a generally widespread and comfortable acceptance of both statements by Canadians. But the last few years, working with colleagues to address vaccine hesitancy and empower individuals with solid scientific information, have challenged my own comfortable assumptions about Canadians' attitudes to science, medicine, public health, and expertise.

I grew up in the UK in an era where an acceptance of and appreciation for science seemed normal and was encouraged. Famous scientists (admittedly almost always white and male) were everywhere, in paintings and statues, in the names of buildings, and were held in the same high regard as artists and composers. Their contributions helped to advance the health and well-being of many. Scientific literacy or, at least, acceptance of the new knowledge gained from the application of scientific methodology was generally seen as a definition of progress. And while scientists are human beings who are deeply flawed in many ways, science is a way of figuring out how the world works, around us and within us. It is a methodology, a process, a set of rules for ensuring that we don't fool ourselves.

Disappointingly, the pandemic has shown me that we are very, very good at fooling ourselves, especially when information doesn't align with our wants and needs and feelings. Some people and organizations will even use a devastating global pandemic as an opportunity to enrich themselves financially and, furthermore, to deliberately delegitimize science for their own ends. The hypocrisy, selfishness, and wilful ignorance on display at the individual and organizational levels have been devastating and depressing. And the business model of creating and amplifying scientific misinformation and disinformation has proven very effective and very lucrative.

I am an academic research scientist trained to make observations, build hypotheses or working models to explain those observations, develop rigorous experimental plans to test those hypotheses or working models, collect and analyse data, and then refine or throw out those models. This is an iterative and collaborative process. There is debate and discourse over those models, but the best ones persist and are continually refined. Sometimes data do not fit the working model, and sometimes something unexpected happens that makes us sit up and think and adjust our underlying assumptions. This is how science works.

In many ways, being a scientist is like being a lawyer and building a case, a compelling case, on the basis of evidence, to convince a jury that, yes, our model is the one that fits the data that we currently have. I love this process. I'm also a vocal supporter of increased science communication and public engagement in Canada. In my role as founding dean of the Faculty of Science at Toronto Metropolitan University, I enthusiastically endorsed and supported Science Rendezvous, a national one-day science fair, where science is celebrated across the country at diverse venues, hosted by local academic institutions. I also brought the award-winning, UK-based program Soapbox Science to Canada, where women from a range of demographics went out on the street to engage with the public about their scientific research, challenging stereotypes and attempting to increase the accessibility of scientific information to the public. My advocacy for making science accessible in Canada is well known.

In the early months of the pandemic, in 2020, there was a flurry of activity among members of the scientific, public health, and medical communities (among others) in terms of ensuring that accurate and comprehensive information about COVID-19 was generated and made widely available to all Canadians. The growing awareness of the dangers of misinformation and disinformation over several months culminated in the formation of ScienceUpFirst, an independent, non-governmental organization whose primary aim would be to provide credible, reliable, and readily accessible information to Canadians, sourced and packaged by teams of independent experts. I was invited to participate in a number of initiatives, among which was joining the executive advisory board of ScienceUpFirst. Initially, the focus of ScienceUpFirst was high-quality, accurate, and easily accessible information about COVID-19–related matters. More recently, ScienceUpFirst staff have expanded their work to cover broader issues of concern to Canadians, such as how to evaluate information peddled by "wellness influencers" on social media; as always, their aim is to help Canadians make accurate, science-informed decisions on their own health and well-being and that of their families.

In the early days of the pandemic, ScienceUpFirst staff worked with social media experts, public health experts, community groups, and others to develop accessible, engaging, and culturally sensitive materials. The particular focus was to engage compassionately and respectfully on common myths about COVID-19 and things like vaccines. The enthusiasm and passion for this work was evident, particularly in young people, many with science backgrounds. All these individuals wanted to participate in a national exercise of knowledge mobilization to make sure Canadians were well informed and could make decisions that would ensure they stayed healthy. These science communicators wanted to make a positive difference with very little in terms of financial compensation. They were doing this because it was the right thing to do and they cared. They looked to successful campaigns over previous decades where outreach and robust science communication about the positive outcomes of vaccinations have led to over 80 per cent of the world's children receiving some sort of protection against previously fatal or disabling infections such as tetanus, whooping cough, measles, and mumps. Astoundingly, the number of children paralyzed by polio has been reduced by 99.9 per cent over the last three decades due to the hard work of healthcare professionals and good quality science communication. An intense plan to eradicate smallpox was launched by the World Health Organization in 1967 and the last natural case was reported in 1977. In a decade, a devastating infection that had plagued humanity for perhaps 3,000 years was eradicated. These were the types of goals that ScienceUpFirst aspired to – help and hope for Canadians in combating and defeating a frightening foe.

In hindsight, this all seems delightfully naive. And perhaps we should have paid more attention, when a colleague pointed out early on, that it's not a lack of information that is really the issue but the ability to distinguish between high-quality, accurate, and scientifically grounded information and misinformation, disinformation, and deliberate lies. Who was telling the truth? And who was lying? And why were they lying? How could the average Canadian tell?

It became increasingly clear that the title of doctor or professor, whether in medicine or science or public health or some other discipline, which would normally be indicative of many years of focused training, was insufficient to ensure that our information was considered trustworthy and reliable.

There has always been a degree of suspicion of the "experts" by some parts of society as a result of systemic patriarchy and racism in science and medicine. Historically, trust in science and medicine has generally been high in Canada. However, we noticed that while there was a lot of positive feedback for the various sources of information and an appreciation for dealing with things like vaccine hesitancy in compassionate, empathetic, and patient ways, there was also a rapidly rising distrust of established institutions and professions in general. We didn't know how to deal with the negative feedback, irrational challenges, and overall scepticism that seemed to be spreading.

As the pandemic dragged on, many of us were dismayed to see colleagues, who were themselves medical doctors and scientists, beginning to make pronouncements that ranged from the weird and ridiculous to the downright dangerous and irresponsible. Why would people do this? Not only did it seem to be a breach of professional standards, it also seemed to be attention-grabbing behaviour, couched in some sort of perverse anti-establishment saviourhood. Challenging orthodoxy was a new badge of honour and the upheaval and anxiety created by the pandemic coupled with social media made for fertile ground for conspiracy theories to flourish, sometimes led by self-described "brave mavericks."

The business model of creating doubt and then selling something, anything (supplements, fake vaccination records, false cures), was amplified. Grift in the industrial wellness complex has always been well established and COVID-19 provided a new name for the problem that could be cured, treated, prevented, and so on if you just signed up and sent money.

Dealing with misinformation and disinformation, particularly on social media, is like cutting off the heads of Hydra. Each time one is removed, two grow back. The sea of misinformation and disinformation is so vast that trying to salvage truth is like "trying to bail out an ocean of water with a teaspoon," to quote American author Jodi Picoult. It is exhausting, depressing, and heart-breaking.

The battle to hold the front lines in telling the truth, presenting the scientific consensus, explaining risk, and explaining scientific process is relentless. The toxic backlash can also, at times, be mentally damaging for those on the front lines. Vitriol from conspiracy theorists and disinformation peddlers is spewed randomly and widely but is also targeted against women, people of colour, and members of the LGBTQ2S+ and other historically marginalized communities. The full range of misogyny, bigotry, hate, and violence has been experienced by everyone trying to communicate legitimate scientific information, but the overwhelming cacophony of abuse has led to my colleagues leaving platforms, locking their accounts, or taking mental health breaks from their roles as science communicators. Dealing with this level of violence, this kind of abuse, is not something that the vast majority of us in science are trained to deal with.

In 2021, the American podcaster Joe Rogan made a number of false statements about COVID-19 vaccines and admitted to taking the anti-parasitic drug ivermectin as a COVID-19 treatment. The structure of his show is well honed and highly successful, and he has found a way to package misinformation and controversy in a very entertaining (to his target demographic) and accessible format by couching his content as "just expressing an opinion." This is a very lucrative business model and Rogan has found the motherlode, with many millions of followers and billions in revenue. When an international collective of scientists, public health experts, and medical professionals asked in a public letter to Spotify, the main platform for Rogan's podcasts, to remove misinformation that could be seriously damaging to public health, the backlash was fast and nasty. As one of the signatories to the letter, I also received emails, which included a missive from the delightful Garry:

> So it appears you have a bone to pick with Joe Rogan.
> You say he's dangerous to public health?
> What a crock of shit lady.
> The only thing dangerous to public health is the bullshit narrative that you spew.
> How dare you.
> You consider yourself an educated woman? Then why not educate yourself.
> You are a pathetic lying coward.
> I'm sure you won't respond to this either ...
> Pathetic coward.

Garry was, at least, less offensive than those sending death and rape threats to my colleagues. Following the release of the Spotify letter, there was also interest from journalists in the story and I was interviewed by a writer for the UK newspaper *The Independent*.[1] The article he wrote had a quote from me, which led to the following email from the charming FB:

> Below is your comment in an *Independent* article in relation to the current hysteria surrounding Joe Rogan and his podcast:
>
> "Falsehoods and misinformation that lead to illness and death (which happens when scientific consensus and public health directives are undermined) surely must be challenged in a free society."
>
> Do you also challenge falsehoods and misinformation when scientific consensus and public health directives are wrong and lead to illness and death? I'd imagine not. You strike me as part of an ever shrinking group of spineless, money hungry, morally corrupt, self-serving, selfish parasites.
>
> Death comes to us all, thankfully. That's one thing not one cunt on this planet can escape. Yet you, and people like you, seem to forget that, and insist on making our lives miserable while you wallow in your vapid, lavish lifestyles.
>
> Reprehensible doesn't even begin to describe it.
>
> We just want to live decent lives for fuck sake.

I'm not sure what a vapid, lavish lifestyle is, but I'm pretty sure I don't have one.

The pandemic has made it crystal clear that far too many in society do not understand how science, as a methodology aimed at preventing us from fooling ourselves, actually works. And we, as scientists and health professionals and science communicators, need to own that failing and double down on our efforts to address that weakness.

Progressive, democratic, inclusive, and healthy societies are scientifically literate societies. It is in our collective interests to ensure the highest levels of scientific literacy, which means explaining science to people. Ed Yong is a brilliant science writer who addressed how science works in his 29 April 2020 article for *The Atlantic*, "Why the Coronavirus Is So Confusing":

> [Science is] less the parade of decisive blockbuster discoveries that the press often portrays, and more a slow, erratic stumble toward ever less uncertainty. "Our understanding oscillates at first, but converges on an answer," says Natalie Dean, a statistician at the University of Florida. "That's the normal scientific process, but it looks jarring to people who aren't used to it."[2]

Here is a take-home lesson for science communicators in Canada: In telling the truth, explain how the truth is determined. Indeed, when I teach critical thinking in the biomedical sciences, I don't ask if you "believe" in the science, or accept as "truth" some sort of statement about vaccines or other biomedical interventions. Beliefs are personal, highly variable, complex, and emotionally rich. Rather, what we should and what we MUST be doing in science communication is explaining that our information comes from the consensus of multiple studies, conducted by diverse scientists in numerous locations over time, that have settled on an explanation for observations and while that explanation is not perfect, based on the body of evidence, it is more likely and plausible than other explanations.

Science communicators must continue to strive for excellence and rigour in their communications while guarding against battle fatigue, cynicism, and despair, which are very real and which grifters and abusers are counting on to silence us. We must redouble our efforts to address the new reality that social media has twisted and corrupted science communication like nothing we have seen before and the reality that social media is providing an opportunity to reach more people in innovative ways than ever before. We need advocacy for more accountability online and activism to tackle the, at times, horrific abuse. We need legislation, regulation, incentivization, and education in a systems-thinking approach to ensure we are all working in the best interests of Canadians' health and well-being using evidence-based, scientifically accurate, and easily accessible information.

It is the consensus, the multitude of asking the questions, all the different ways, by different people, and building that understanding, in a slow and erratic way, staggering towards less and less uncertainty. It's not pretty, or easy, and doesn't result in most of us (scientists, clinicians, public health professionals) getting rich (and supporting our vapid lifestyles!). But importantly, it works in terms of preventing us from fooling ourselves. In theory, it should also help us fight off grifters and hucksters. *Caveat emptor!*

The pandemic has seen an increase in spread and acceptance of conspiracy theories, an alarming increase in the abuse of professionals in science, public health, and medicine, and a coordinated attack on the institutions and processes that protect us. Where are we heading, Canada?

IMOGEN R. COE, MSC, PHD, is the founding dean of the Faculty of Science, Toronto Metropolitan University; an affiliate scientist at the Li Ka Shing Knowledge Institute, Keenan Research Centre, St. Michael's Hospital; past-president (2020–2) of the Canadian Society for Molecular Biosciences; a member of the board at Michael Garron Hospital; and a member of the Executive Advisory Committee at ScienceUpFirst.

I Work in a Hospital.
You Are an Internet Troll.
We Are Not the Same

DR. GENEVIEVE EASTABROOK

"Thirteen stillbirths in a 24-hour period at Lions Gate Hospital" was the outlandish claim made in late 2021 by two physicians who believed that COVID-19 was a hoax, and that the mRNA vaccines were causing stillbirth, disability, and death.[1] This disinformation campaign spread rapidly online, with similar claims cropping up in several other cities. It got so bad that several health authorities and hospital networks had to put out press releases stating that these claims were unequivocally false. Nonetheless, pregnant people hearing these claims were terrified – even those who had received vaccines prior to becoming pregnant. This was a concern that prevented several of my patients from receiving second or third doses.

Earlier in 2021, I received a referral for a patient who had already fired two obstetricians. The note from the family physician read, "Please don't discuss COVID vaccines

whatsoever." I started with a phone consultation with
Skye,[2] who didn't want to come to the hospital for her appointment because she was concerned about vaccine shed-
ding. After many gentle conversations, I was finally able to
convince her to come and see me in person. Skye arrived
with a detailed care plan, which laid bare her vaccine-
related anxiety, including her concerns that we would vac-
cinate both her and her baby without their consent. She was
also adamant that she would refuse a medically necessary
blood transfusion, as she believed that the blood may contain "vaccine contaminated" blood. After reading so many
internet posts from people saying that those of us who supported COVID-19 protection measures were "living in fear,"
here was a person willing to jeopardize her own health and
the outcome of her pregnancy because she was afraid of
the COVID-19 vaccine. She'd gone months without an in-
person prenatal visit and ended up contracting COVID-19 a
few weeks before our first meeting. Despite being hospitalized, she still believed that the vaccine was worse than the
disease.

I have learned that there is a small percentage of vaccine-
hesitant people who will never change their stance, regardless of being bombarded with good quality information
from peers or experts. Skye was one of those people. During our appointments, I did not discuss COVID-19 vaccines
whatsoever because I didn't want her to flee from my care
and end up with a catastrophic complication while attempting an unaccompanied birth in her remote home, something
she said she had considered. Ultimately, the outcome was
good: she had a healthy baby and left the hospital as soon

as humanly possible. I think of Skye often, her wide, frightened eyes pleading with me to understand where she was coming from. How did she get to that point? Where did her fears begin? Who had lied to her in such a compelling way that she was willing to sacrifice her life? I am not angry at Skye, or the many pregnant people like her. I am angry at those who peddle disinformation that frightens vulnerable people to such a degree that they hurt themselves, and sometimes others.

It is now common knowledge that there are massive, well-coordinated online disinformation campaigns that politicize and undermine confidence in vaccines, masks, and other pandemic mitigation measures. These were more than just the few grifters preying on "natural parenting" groups that I had grown used to tackling. Whenever I posted anything about COVID-19 vaccines, especially in the context of pregnancy, my Twitter account was swarmed by trolls.

I have existed as a woman on the internet (and in medicine) for a long time, and therefore have a very thick skin, but I had never experienced an outpouring of vitriol and ad hominem attacks to this extent, even on posts related to other controversial topics, such as abortion access or transgender rights. While some were "real" people, many were obvious bots or sock puppet accounts. Like many physicians active on social media during the pandemic, I have been threatened with being put on trial for crimes against humanity ("Nuremberg 2.0"), had my credentials questioned, and been called a lizard person, a witch, and a pedophile. My usual tactic is simply to ignore and block these accounts, unless they are making threats, in which case I report them first. Occasionally, I will retort with a comment, such as "I work in a hospital. You are an internet troll. We are not the same." A couple of months ago, one of my patients presented me with a custom-made T-shirt with this phrase printed on the front. I was delighted, both by the thoughtful gesture and that my presence on social media may be making a meaningful difference in vaccine confidence and uptake.

For more than a decade on Twitter, I have shared accurate and accessible health information, especially about pregnancy, birth, and parenting. Vaccines, and vaccine hesitancy, are a particular area of interest: I studied immunology during my undergraduate degree and went on to do research in the immunology of placental formation as both an OBGYN resident and a maternal fetal medicine fellow. I came of age in the era where vaccine hesitancy reared its ugly head, around the time of Andrew Wakefield's falsified study wrongly implicating the MMR vaccine in causing autism. Having both a sibling and a child with autism, shutting down vaccine disinformation, especially the ableist and eugenicist aspects of this ideology, is both a personal and a professional mission. I also really, really detest watching people become ill from vaccine-preventable illnesses because they have been lied to by charlatans trying to sell "natural" cures, including potentially toxic products like the anti-parasitic drug ivermectin or homeopathic remedies that are essentially water.

Prior to the pandemic, I had always made a point of sharing on social media that my entire family had received influenza vaccines and reminding pregnant people to get theirs. In my high-risk OB clinic, vaccine uptake is typically higher than in a low-risk pregnancy population, particularly after I've counselled people regarding the benefits to both themselves and their babies of being protected against the flu and its complications. Invariably, there were always internet trolls who made spurious claims about vaccines being unsafe in pregnancy, calling me a "big pharma shill," but these were tame in comparison with what was to come with the roll out of the COVID-19 mRNA vaccines.

In addition to malignant campaigns of disinformation, there is a systemic issue in perinatal health that underlies much of this suspicion and fear: pregnant people, and women in general, have been excluded from pharmaceutical trials for decades. Thus, there is no good counterargument when people say, "But there is no data in pregnancy!" Sadly, this is by design. Pregnancy, or even the possibility that one could become pregnant, is an exclusion criterion for most drug trials, including for vaccines. Many potentially life-saving treatments for critically ill people also lack pregnancy-specific data.

Perhaps one positive outcome of this pandemic has been the increased public awareness that pregnant people and women of reproductive age are excluded and/or underrepresented in clinical research. This has led to calls for action by ethicists, scientists, and patients themselves, demanding that patient autonomy and informed choice be respected so that pregnant people and women of reproductive age can choose to be included in pharmaceutical studies.

Around the time that the first COVID-19 mRNA vaccines became available, I was asked by one of the ICU consultants to give a talk on COVID-19 vaccination in pregnancy to their staff. Despite the increasingly worrisome data around COVID-19 in pregnancy, there was significant vaccine hesitancy, even among the nurses and other staff working with COVID-19 positive patients in the ICU. I began to worry in earnest about vaccine uptake: If pregnant healthcare workers in the highest risk environments were more worried about vaccine side effects than COVID-19 itself, what hope was there for everyone else?

The initial reassurances that pregnant people would not experience worse outcomes from COVID-19 than anyone else were short-lived, particularly as Delta became the dominant variant. Maria, a pregnant nurse on the respirology unit, broke down during one of her clinic appointments with me after disclosing that she was told that her use of an N95 mask during her shifts was "inappropriate" despite caring for COVID-19 positive patients. She had only received one dose of COVID-19 vaccine at this point. I wrote a note advising her superiors that she would have to remain off work for the remainder of her pregnancy, citing insufficient accommodations for a high-risk medical condition. She was plagued with guilt for leaving her unit short-staffed, but she had no other safe choice.

We now know that pregnancy is an independent risk factor for severe morbidity and death from COVID-19, especially in unvaccinated individuals. Whether it was because of a high vaccine uptake and a fairly high rate of compliance with pandemic protections, the centre where I work had only a handful of pregnant people admitted to the intensive care unit for COVID-19 and its complications. Before COVID-19, having a pregnant or postpartum patient die was a rare event that shook our entire department. And yet, after the COVID-19 Delta wave, we felt thankful for only two maternal deaths. Among the other very sick, unvaccinated pregnant patients, there were stillbirths, preterm births, and neonatal deaths. Some survivors and their families later expressed regret at not getting vaccinated, but many others were steadfast in their convictions that the illness that took the lives of their partners, daughters, or babies was simply "a flu" or something that would have happened anyway.

The gulf between vaccine opinions in pregnant people is enormous. I've cared for triple-vaccinated healthcare workers, teachers, and other essential workers who worry about the impact of breakthrough infections on the developmental outcomes of their babies and who were willing to travel out of province or even to the United States before fourth doses were available in Ontario. I've also cared for medically complex and immunocompromised women, facing major surgery, who have had only one dose pre-pregnancy and are now terrified to receive further vaccines while pregnant because they "read that there were more than 30 stillbirths in Hamilton linked to the vaccine."[3] Jasmine, a cancer survivor, told me that she hadn't completely ruled out receiving the COVID-19 vaccine during her pregnancy, but that she was "just waiting to hear about it from an expert source." After gently reminding her that I *was* an expert source, she went home to discuss things further with her husband. At the next visit, she told me that while she was open to the vaccine, her husband didn't want her to receive it until after the baby was born. I told her, "I hope you know that this is your choice and not his. He doesn't even have to know."

I don't know what Jasmine eventually decided, but I was glad that we were able to have this conversation. I will keep having these conversations, whether in person or online, for as long as they are needed.

DR. EASTABROOK is an associate professor of OBGYN and a maternal fetal medicine subspecialist at the University of Western Ontario. She is a clinician-researcher and co-lead of Western's Pregnancy Research Group (PRG).

How to Be Wrong: Reflections on the (Non)Evolution of Applied Medical Science during Epidemics

DR. DAVID FISMAN

A Global Catastrophe, in Retrospect

A pandemic of SARS-2 coronavirus (COVID-19), a novel disease that emerged globally in January 2020, has killed close to 7 million people globally at the time of writing;[1] accounting for under-reporting, the true death toll is likely to have been something like 26 million.[2] The pandemic has exacerbated economic inequality,[3] has orphaned millions of children,[4] and may be increasing risk for cardiac disease,[5] as well as neurodevelopmental delay in infants.[6] In short, this pandemic has been a global catastrophe, despite rapid development of vaccines,[7] the availability of accurate tests,[8] and early identification of the dominant aerosol transmission of the pathogen.[9]

Available tools should have reduced the global death toll, as is clear when differences in cumulative mortality

Figure 26.1. Cumulative COVID-19 mortality as of 12 October 2022.

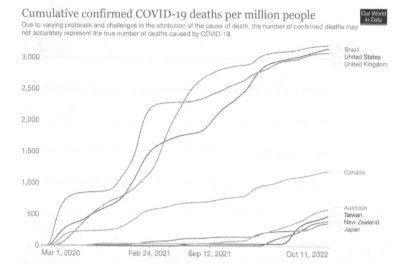

Cumulative confirmed COVID-19 deaths per million people

Due to varying protocols and challenges in the attribution of the cause of death, the number of confirmed deaths may not accurately represent the true number of deaths caused by COVID-19.

Our World in Data (Open Access), https://ourworldindata.org
/coronavirus#explore-the-global-situation
Notes: Clear qualitative differences are seen in cumulative deaths over the first thirty-three months of the global SARS-CoV-2 pandemic between countries that used available tools with a goal of elimination early in the pandemic (Japan, Taiwan, New Zealand, and Australia), and countries that engaged in modest mitigation efforts (Brazil, United States, United Kingdom). The outcome of the Canadian response is intermediate between these two groupings.

between countries that aggressively applied control measures early in the pandemic and those that did not are compared (Figure 26.1).[10]

The fact that millions of deaths could have been prevented, but were not, should serve as a starting point for any attempt to learn from the pandemic. Learning the lessons of the pandemic will not bring back the dead, but understanding what happened is important for two reasons. First, tools that might have substantially mitigated the spread of SARS-CoV-2 are still underused in the face of what is now a highly virulent endemic disease. Second, the emergence of new highly transmissible viruses with pandemic potential is likely in the future. Most viruses with pandemic potential appear at the "human-animal interface": the contact point between humans and animals in the wild, in food markets and food production facilities, and in laboratories. Ongoing environmental degradation, industrial food production practices,[11] and risky research[12] also make it likely that many of us will experience another pandemic in our lifetimes.

To understand what has happened over the last few years, and to address future pandemics, we must understand and learn from history. In the next few pages, I will discuss the ongoing failure by many organizations and individual scientists to acknowledge dominant aerosol transmission of SARS-CoV-2[13] as a signal failure of the pandemic public health response. This failure is by no means specific to the SARS-CoV-2 pandemic, as the cholera pandemics of the nineteenth century illustrate. I will discuss the role of uncertainty, including manufactured uncertainty and disinformation, in slowing effective action. I will argue that the suboptimal control of this disease was less reflective of scientific uncertainty and more about a lack of consensus around values, or perhaps more accurately, a gap between values endorsed publicly by decision-makers, and those held (and acted on) more privately.

Past as Prologue: Nineteenth-Century Debates on Cholera and Miasma

Past pandemics have much to teach us: they tell us that scientific truth isn't enough to instantaneously change policy, but that understanding the mode of transmission of diseases is central to their control.

Cholera, a virulent diarrhoeal disease resulting from bacterial infection, endemic to the Ganges River Delta, emerged as a global pandemic threat in the early nineteenth century. By the 1820s, cholera epidemics were described in Central Asia, along the route of the Old Silk Road, and the disease emerged in Russia by 1829.[14] Initially perceived as a communicable threat, Russian authorities attempted to prevent movement of the disease by establishing a military *cordon sanitaire* (literally a "rope of health," which was a blockade consisting of roadblocks to prevent movement of people and goods). The blockade failed to prevent the spread of cholera, presumably as a result of the blockade being leaky and because of contamination of water sources that crossed the blockade, but it did cause an economic and civil crisis in Saint Petersburg.[15] The Russian experience suggested to decision-makers that the disease might not be communicable, or in any case, that a high price could be paid by treating it as though it was.[16] The concept of miasma (a poisonous gas that spread disease) was not new, but had been bolstered by early nineteenth-century French studies that showed the risk of disease to be correlated with filth and foul odours.[17] This provided a ready conceptual model for miasmatic transmission of cholera.[18]

Data collected when cholera emerged in New York State in 1832 are clearly supportive of the communicability of cholera, which arrived sequentially in towns by moving along the major transportation arteries of the day.[19] Nonetheless, these data were used to argue for the miasmatic (non-communicable) nature of this disease. The poor moral constitution, or sinful behaviour, of individuals stricken with cholera was invoked to explain the uneven distribution of the disease, effectively changing the focus of prevention from the level of society (trade, travel, and commerce) to individuals.[20]

The treatment of foul odours as agents of disease directly informed public policy, with English sanitarians leading a successful campaign for construction of sewers in London by the late 1840s, to remove foul smells from neighbourhoods by piping waste into the River Thames.[21] The River Thames provided drinking water to the city. Viewed from a twenty-first-century vantage point, investment in sewers that *facilitated* the mixing of sewage and drinking water seems absurd, but it was entirely reasonable under the prevailing miasmatic disease transmission model. Sewage contamination of drinking water resulted in large cholera epidemics in London in the early 1850s.

While the prevailing establishment view held that cholera was non-contagious, a contrary view was held by the early anaesthetist John Snow.[22] Snow was uniquely positioned to be an outsider: his work as the anaesthetist to Queen Victoria had made him independently wealthy.[23] In his studies of anaesthesia, he had become familiar with gas laws described by early nineteenth-century French chemists.[24]

Snow saw that patterns of cholera death were inconsistent with the expected behaviour of a gas.[25] He also intuited that gastrointestinal symptoms suggested an ingested agent, and noted less disease in brewers, who tended to drink beer rather than water.[26] His linkage of cholera to travellers allowed him to focus on humans rather than the environment.[27] Snow's basic argument was in print by 1849,[28] but it was seven years from the initial publication of his pamphlet to its endorsement by London's General Board of Health (1856).[29] The magnitude and frequency of cholera epidemics declined in the United States and the United Kingdom once an identification of the mode of transmission allowed implementation of effective preventive measures.[30] Success in the control of cholera in high-income countries should have served to demonstrate the centrality of understanding disease transmission for control.

Snow's refutation of the theory of miasmas, and the subsequent recognition of the centrality of microbes in the transmission of communicable diseases, informed the ideas of American physician-epidemiologist Charles Chapin, who conceptualized respiratory disease as being spread at short range by moist respiratory droplets. Chapin's statement that infections are spread by contact and are "sprayborne for only two or three feet" was accepted as gospel for the next 110 years.[31] While Chapin lacked the technical resources to characterize respiratory aerosols, other researchers like Mildred and William Wells and Richard Riley had accurately described the physics and behaviour of small respiratory particles by 1934.[32] Aerosols are tiny particles suspended in a gas; aerosol behaviour occurs when such particles are smaller than 100 micrometres in diameter. In the context of communicable diseases, that gas is the atmosphere that we breathe;[33] one familiar example of an aerosol is cigarette smoke. Although we perceive smoke as a "cloud," it actually consists of tiny particles suspended in air. The extremely small size of aerosol particles means that they don't fall immediately to the ground due to gravity but can drift and float for considerable periods of time and can distribute themselves throughout a closed indoor environment (again, one can visualize cigarette smoke hanging in the lights in an old-time club, even after the patrons have gone home). Abundant respiratory aerosols are produced by breathing, talking, shouting, and coughing.[34]

William Wells and Riley validated their work by demonstrating the airborne transmission of tuberculosis, via respiratory aerosols from infected patients, in hospital environments,[35] but influential figures in the public health establishment remained loyal to Chapin's incorrect model, even creating parallel physical models rooted in error,[36] in which aerosol behaviour is attributed only to particles smaller than 5 μm in diameter and considered to be the property of individual pathogens themselves. Mid-sized respiratory aerosol particles are thousands of times larger (by volume) than bacteria, and hundreds of thousands of times larger than viruses. There is no reason to expect that the ability to be carried in aerosol is restricted to a limited number of specific respiratory pathogens. In medicine, however, pathogens such as measles, varicella, and smallpox have been admitted into this exclusive aerosol "club" on a case-by-case basis, following extraordinary outbreaks that made spread by any other route implausible.[37]

Wrongness and Aerosol Transmission of Viral Respiratory Disease: A Case Study

Characteristics of aerosols that are important for communicable disease spread include their generation by quiet breathing and talking (so that disease can be transmitted by individuals without symptoms), and their ability to "float" for a considerable period of time in room air. A high-to-low concentration gradient with distance from the source patient predicts that infection at close range will be more common than infection at longer range.[38]

At the time of the emergence of the SARS-CoV-2 pandemic, dominant medical dogma held that most respiratory diseases are transmitted by "droplets" or direct contact, representing a direct application of Chapin's ideas from the early twentieth century. This erroneous information with no basis in physical reality was codified in public health and hospital infection control guidance, which was still available on the internet as of October 2022,[39] and which was invoked during the pandemic. The distinction is important: acknowledging aerosol transmission leads directly to identification of existing preventive measures, which can be categorized broadly as ventilation, filtration (either using air filters, or by using properly fitting respirator masks), and disinfection using high-room UV radiation.[40] As infective aerosols are generated by individuals with or without symptoms, masks are also useful as source control.

Early in the pandemic, high attack rates among Chinese healthcare workers led health authorities in China to

Figure 26.2. *Text of factually incorrect tweet by the World Health Organization, stating that SARS-CoV-2 is not airborne.*

FACT: #COVID19 is NOT airborne.

The #coronavirus is mainly transmitted through droplets generated when an infected person coughs, sneezes or speaks.

To protect yourself:
- keep 1m distance from others
- disinfect surfaces frequently
- wash/rub your [hands emoji]
- avoid touching your [eyes emoji] [nose emoji] [mouth emoji]

The tweet was sent on 28 March 2020, and despite an abundance of evidence demonstrating it to be false, it remains publicly available at https://mobile.twitter.com/WHO/status/1243972193169616898 as of 12 October 2022.

mandate the use of N95 masks, which resulted in a dramatic reduction in infection risk.[41] A paper using Chinese contact data from January and February 2020 strongly suggested that aerosol transmission was present.[42] Further data supporting aerosol transmission accumulated rapidly.[43]

Nonetheless, major public health and infection control authorities continued to dismiss the idea that the pandemic was transmitted via respiratory aerosols. The World Health Organization (WHO) infamously stated "Fact: #COVID19 is NOT airborne" in a posting on Twitter. That tweet was uncorrected and not retracted as of October 2022 (Figure 26.2). An open letter by prominent aerosol scientists to the WHO urging the use of aerosol science to control the pandemic[44] resulted in little action and was met with a dismissive response by numerous Canadian infection control physicians.[45]

Would Correctly Identifying the Dominant Mode of SARS-CoV-2 Transmission Have Made Any Difference?

Did failure to act on dominant airborne transmission change the trajectory of the pandemic? The answer is clearly "yes." In order to understand why, we need to understand the concept of a "basic reproduction number" (R_0) of a communicable disease. The R_0 is the number of new infections created by an infectious case in a population with no immunity, and without any disease control interventions in place. For example, if the R_0 for a disease was 3, we would expect an infected case to create 3 new cases before recovery or death; each of those 3 cases would create 3 new cases (9 in total), which in turn would create 3 new cases (27 in total), and so on. The number of cases in this simple example is increasing exponentially with time; it's an epidemic. Epidemic spread occurs when the basic reproduction number (R_0) of a pathogen is greater than 1.

Let's consider SARS-CoV-2. That virus had an initial R_0 around 2.2.[46] R_0 is proportional to the number of contacts the case has per day, the probability that the case infects each of those contacts, and the length of time the case is infectious. For example, if people have 3 contacts per day, they infect (on average) 37 per cent of the cases they contact, and are infectious for

2 days, you'd expect an R_0 of 2.2 (3 x 0.37 x 2 = 2.2). Reducing any one of these components of R_0 (infectivity, contact numbers, or duration of infectivity) reduces R proportionately.[47] Now consider that, as demonstrated later in the pandemic, improvements in ventilation reduced transmission by 40 per cent,[48] while use of fitted respirators reduced transmission by 80 per cent.[49] Such interventions would have been expected to reduce an R_0 of 2.2 to 0.26; that would have been enough to cause SARS-CoV-2 to go extinct (be eradicated, in epidemiological terms), as was achieved with SARS-CoV-1.

Instead, muddled messaging on mode of transmission and mask efficacy[50] allowed global exponential growth in case counts. Over time this made elimination far more challenging, and ultimately impossible. Health authorities demanded scientific certainty before taking action, which goes against the "precautionary principle," which states that "complete evidence of a potential risk is not required before action is taken to mitigate the effects of the … risk."[51] The virus mutated and adapted due to hundreds of millions of transmissions in humans, creating more transmissible and immunity-evading variants.[52] The virus was able to recross the barrier between humans and animal species,[53] creating animal reservoirs that make it impossible to push SARS-CoV-2 to extinction (be eradicated). The failure of health authorities to apply existing tools for the control of an airborne disease resulted in worse global health outcomes and in higher economic costs for everyone. This failure is reminiscent of failures of reasoning encountered during the cholera pandemics of the nineteenth century, and I suspect will be remembered similarly. The parallels between these pandemics are outlined in Box 26.1.

Box 26.1. Parallel reasons for failing to accept dominant airborne transmission of SARS-CoV-2 and contagiousness of cholera in the nineteenth century.

1. **Fidelity to outdated mental models of disease transmission, and/or inability or unwillingness to assimilate emerging scientific data.**

    a. Cholera: Unfamiliarity of Sanitarians with gas laws, which made miasmatic spread implausible.

    b. SARS-CoV-2: Lack of familiarity among the public health and infectious disease communities with body of knowledge related to behaviour of aerosols. Fidelity to an outdated medical canon (e.g., Chapin's model).

2. **Workload or resource implications of acknowledging error.**

    a. Cholera: Need to find alternate, non-contaminated water sources in the nineteenth century. Need to alter major infrastructure projects built based on input from Sanitarian community.

    b. SARS-CoV-2: Challenges in managing airborne disease in healthcare with current limitations of physical resources (ventilation and filtration constraints in hospitals, lack of negative pressure isolation rooms, multibed rooms in hospitals become problematic); need for employers and landlords to improve ventilation in workplaces and apartment buildings; need to revise infection control guidance.

3. **Embarrassment or shame at having to admit error.**

4. **Change in locus of responsibility for infection preven-tion from individuals to institutions, which would need to provide clean, safe environments.**

   a. Cholera: Can no longer blame cholera victims for infec-tion caused by weak moral constitutions. Obligation of governments and companies to provide clean drinking water to citizens and customers.

   b. SARS-CoV-2: Can no longer blame SARS-CoV-2 victims for infection caused by donning/doffing of personal protective equipment or social activities when not in the workplace or public spaces. Obligation of govern-ments and companies to provide clean air, with impli-cations for liability and costs if they fail to do so.

Uncertainty, Manufactured Uncertainty, and Disinformation

While science provides the knowledge base that is used to inform decisions about communicable disease control, those decisions are often made by political actors, using policy levers. During my time as a member of Ontario's "COVID Science Table," expert guidance from (arguably) the prov-ince's top scientists passed through a filter of elected pol-iticians. While this is how we would expect a democracy to function, the resultant governmental guidance often failed to prioritize population health, while this process simultaneously allowed politicians to state that they were "following the science." In his book on relationships between scientists and policymakers, *The Honest Broker*, political scientist Roger Pielke[54] notes that science-based policy decisions are often "hard" when there is disagreement on values and/or when there is important scientific uncertainty. When these conditions are not present the scientist can simply play a translational role (as a "science arbiter," to use Pielke's term).[55]

However, the role of the scientist is more challenging when there is a lack of consensus on values, or when there is substantial scientific uncertainty. Roger Pielke notes, insightfully, that "[u]ncertainty is ... a resource for various interests in the process of bargaining, negotiation, and compromise." His characterization of science-informed policymaking as heavily influenced by two basic domains, values consensus and scientific uncertainty,[56] can provide insights into how decisions were made during the pandemic.

The emphasis on values acknowledges that disease control programs may have multiple, competing objectives. For example, while a public values consensus might suggest that the primary objective of the pandemic response was protection of the population's health, the reality was more complex. Across jurisdictions, objectives of SARS-CoV-2 control programs might include prevention of death, preservation of health systems, maintenance of educational systems, protection of economies or specific sectors within economies (the restaurant industry, for example), and so on. This is not new, and the utilitarian ethical frame commonly applied in public health and medicine can accommodate competing objectives. In a utilitarian frame, policies are considered optimal if they provide the greatest good for the greatest number, at a reasonable cost.[57]

I would argue, however, that while there has been some scientific uncertainty during the pandemic, the precautionary principle would have been invoked *if values consensus had truly been present* (Figure 26.3). Furthermore, as noted above, many of the hallmarks of SARS-CoV-2 that provided a roadmap for an effective pandemic response were available by the spring of 2020. In the face of little important uncertainty, and values consensus, it should have been possible for scientists to advise optimal action as in Figure 26.3. Indeed, countries that explicitly attempted to eliminate SARS-CoV-2 had fewer deaths, less mental health impacts, and *less* stringent pandemic responses over time than those that simply aimed for mitigation.[58]

It is my opinion that the reason many Western countries struggled to respond to the SARS-CoV-2 pandemic was not because they lacked information but because leaders and other people of influence had different priorities than those that they publicly endorsed. Early aggressive pandemic responses were associated with declines in financial markets (though whether these declines reflected control measures, the pandemic itself, or some combination is unclear),[59] while acceptance of aerosol transmission to make workplaces and school environments safe would have shifted the responsibility for disease and death to governments, healthcare facilities, and employers, which would result in costs to them in the near term (but might be expected to reduce illness-related costs in the longer term). Consultants working for Western governments on pandemic responses may have also had important conflicts of interest related to pandemic policies.[60] It was hard, politically, to explain these different priorities publicly, and I believe that it was in this context that scientific uncertainty was manufactured, where little existed, including via disinformation campaigns that have been a hallmark of the pandemic.[61]

Preferred policies that reflected the values consensus of those in power, but not society more broadly, may have *excluded* equitable protection of life and health. In this context, alternative objectives more amenable to a broad values consensus (for example, possible impacts of school closures on children's mental health) but favouring predetermined policy actions (e.g., "a return to normal") were emphasized to the exclusion of all else, despite considerable evidentiary uncertainty around negative effects of school closures on children's mental health during the pandemic (as opposed to whether changes represented a continuation of phenomena that preceded the pandemic).[62] This creation of uncertainty (whether by disinformation, by dismantling surveillance systems, or by making data unavailable to the public), and the need to put forward alternative consensus values that could win public support to pursue predetermined policies, is illustrated schematically in Figure 26.3.

Pielke suggests that scientific decision-making is defined by the presence or absence of values consensus and scientific uncertainty. On the two-dimensional plane, values consensus (up = increasing) is represented on the vertical axis, while scientific uncertainty (rightward = increasing) is represented on the horizontal axis. When there is large

Figure 26.3. *Schema proposing roles of values consensus and scientific uncertainty in pandemic decision-making, adapted from Roger Pielke,* **The Honest Broker** *(2007), 58, 59. © David Fisman.*

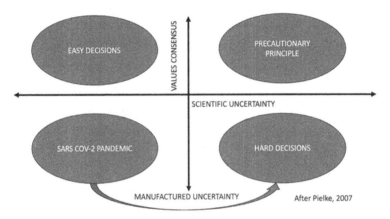

scientific uncertainty, but a clear values consensus (top right), policy may be formulated, and action taken, based on the precautionary principle. When there is little scientific uncertainty, and values consensus (top left), optimal policy should be straightforward. At bottom left, there is little scientific uncertainty, but values consensus is lacking. The desired policies of influential stakeholders may in fact run counter to broader societal values; successful implementation of policy requires emphasis of an acceptable values consensus, with the manufacture of uncertainty creating "space for negotiation," to use Pielke's term. Uncertainty can be manufactured through the generation of disinformation, by dismantling surveillance systems, or by making data unavailable to the public.

Challenges for Twenty-First-Century Public Health

The global SARS-CoV-2 pandemic has been a catastrophe for human health and is likely to have health and economic consequences that reverberate for decades to come. The poignancy of this tragedy is heightened by the fact that a far earlier, and far more effective, public health response could have been supported by early data that demonstrated airborne transmission of SARS-CoV-2. The non-application of these tools in a timely way allowed space for viral evolution, as well as the establishment of infection in non-human animal populations (i.e., zoonotic reservoirs), ensuring that SARS-CoV-2 will remain a human health challenge for the foreseeable future.

The numerous parallels between the nineteenth-century responses to cholera pandemics and the twenty-first-century responses to SARS-CoV-2 suggest that dysfunctional responses of organizations and hierarchies to novel communicable disease threats transcend time, place, and the specific features of an individual disease. Misalignment of the values and objectives of influential individuals and groups, and the implications of moving culpability for disease spread from private individuals to governments and institutions, likely delayed responses to public health crises during both pandemics.

In a sense, the availability of sophisticated disinformation, amplified by social media, makes the challenges for the twenty-first century even greater than they were for the nineteenth. Greater awareness of how disinformation can distort pandemic responses is an important area of focus for future pandemics, and a more ecumenical, and less rigid, understanding of the sources and meanings of scientific evidence may allow improved responses to future epidemics and pandemics.[63] Understanding the dynamics of interactions between morality, altruism, and self-interest, which may underpin public health decision-making, is likely an important area for study, and one that is already being examined by behavioural economists.[64]

Ultimately, however, the challenges of the SARS-CoV-2 pandemic have their roots not in scientific uncertainty or the absence of tools for disease control but in the lack of values consensus, and in the disconnections between which values are endorsed publicly by decision-makers and which determine policymaking. While there is great interest in the limitations and failures of health systems during the pandemic, emerging evidence suggests that the SARS-CoV-2 mortality risk in Canada may have been driven more by upstream factors, such as interactions between race, poverty, and living conditions, than by access to healthcare.[65] The ability of individuals to limit exposure to a disease spread through shared air in schools, workplaces, and apartment buildings is limited. This points to a new emphasis on safe, clean indoor air as a paradigm shift that will increase health equity in the aftermath of the pandemic. This approach would represent a twenty-first century parallel with successful late nineteenth-century and early twentieth-century efforts to prevent cholera and other waterborne diseases. Notably, indoor air can be made cleaner and safer using relatively inexpensive tools (such as filtration and high-room UV radiation) that have existed for decades.[66] Innovation is often held up as the cure-all for future infectious disease crises, but our failure to use existing tools during the current pandemic suggests that our challenges are more political than scientific.

Acknowledgments

Ideas discussed in this chapter owe much to presentations at the University of Michigan, the European Working Group on Surveillance of Influenza, and the University of Toronto Engineering and Psychology Seminars, as well as to discussions with Drs. Michael Fisman, Malgorzata Gasperowicz, Trish Greenhalgh, Jose Luis Jimenez, Linsey Marr, Kimberly Prather, and Ashleigh Tuite.

DR. FISMAN is a physician-epidemiologist with research interests that fall at the intersection of applied epidemiology, mathematical modelling, and applied health economics. He trained in medicine and epidemiology at Western, McGill, Brown, and Harvard universities, and has held faculty appointments at Drexel, McMaster, Princeton, and the University of Toronto, where he is currently professor of epidemiology. During the SARS-CoV-2 pandemic he served on both national and provincial advisory groups, and held emergency COVID-19 research funds from the Canadian Institutes of Health Research. He leads the Pandemic Readiness stream at the recently founded University of Toronto Institute for Pandemics.

Postscript: Roll Up Your Sleeves

SUE ROBINS

Dear Readers:

I want to leave you with hope. Not pseudo-hope that is steeped in denial, but hope that is real.

During the pandemic, my own hope has become deeply intertwined with despair. Since March 2020, I have learned that hope and despair can actually co-exist on the same day or even in the same moment. Hope does not mean that everything will be okay. Hope means waking up to try for a better day.

The authors in this book have passionately laid out that the world has irrevocably changed since the pandemic arrived at our doorstep. *Breaking Canadians* is a unique and timely telling of our pandemic stories from people with diverse perspectives: nurses, physicians, researchers, caregivers, teachers, and disabled people, including those living with long COVID.

The people who make decisions in our healthcare systems, including the executives who are responsible for the lack of public health policies, have harmed all of us in some way. Our healing begins when we dare to share our stories about these harms.

Kudos to the writers for revisiting some of the most excruciating times of their lives for this book. They have shone light on their pain so that we can learn from their wisdom. This book includes a spectrum of experiences that are equally important: stories of staff in moral distress working in long-term care, caregivers struggling at home, and patients enduring cruel and unsafe healthcare settings. Maggie Keresteci describes with eloquent sorrow the fact that we are not in this together after all. The betrayal of society and governments that have failed to protect immune-compromised people like Maggie's family members – and my own disabled son – is deep and painful.

This trauma will not soon be forgotten and many of us will live for the rest of our lives with the effects of the government's lack of response to the pandemic.

This book touches on many emotions from the past years: fury, sorrow, distress, exhaustion, despair, impatience, and disappointment. Underpinning most of these emotions? Fear. This pandemic has suspended me in fear for more than three years. I've never felt such unrelenting fear of my own mortality, even when I was a cancer patient. It is difficult to even take a breath in the midst of such crushing terror. We must keep breathing to continue on. One step at a time; one breath at a time.

The writers in this book are fully standing in their own truth. These people are courageous truth-tellers. Courage means being afraid and doing it anyway. Speaking up is risky in Canada, a place that believes in the myth of its perfect health system. Offering constructive feedback about healthcare is frowned on. To paraphrase health journalist André Picard, Canadians offer themselves cold comfort by saying it's a lot worse in the United States.

Dr. Brian Goldman opens *Breaking Canadians* with the assertion that the path forward is empathy. There's a difference between thinking that you care and actually doing something to demonstrate caring. It is now time to demonstrate action.

It is past time for the people of Canada to speak up. Don't wait until you are a patient, for then you may be too sick to act. Write your government officials. Research healthcare approaches used in other countries. Organize over your virtual kitchen tables. Support each other emotionally. Send a food delivery to a sick colleague. Shout – loudly when needed – on social media. Join a demonstration at the legislature to support public healthcare. Pick up medication from the pharmacy for your neighbour. Reject tone policing from those who want to shut you up.

Importantly, make the time to write a letter of gratitude to those who care for you and your loved ones. I'm grateful to Dr. Nili Kaplan-Myrth for leading the charge with *Breaking Canadians*. I'm thankful for the beautifully diverse writers in this book. My hope is that turning the randomness of the pandemic into a story helped each contributor make sense of an impossible situation and set them on the road to healing. For me, I feel a little less lonely and broken after reading this book.

Breaking Canadians is the book we need right now. Do not turn away from the suffering. Looking at our own mortality squarely in the face can bond us patients and clinicians together as human beings. Above all else, we all need to be more human right now.

Ultimately, my hope does not come from politicians or health officials. My hope comes from the advocacy demonstrated by the people in *Breaking Canadians*. Some of us have been advocating for improving Canada's health system for a long time, while others are new to activism.

Let's welcome other healthcare advocates with open arms. This can be demoralizing, dangerous, and frustrating work. Those embedded within the establishment do not appreciate those of us who rail against the status quo. It helps to know we aren't alone. If this book serves to connect these scattered advocates through their words, then that's a job well done. Every revolution starts with a conversation. May this book spark these conversations.

If you read this book and weep, take that sorrow and turn it into action. Since this book was written, the situation in paediatric healthcare has become even more dire. Children are falling ill and dying from COVID-19, influenza, and respiratory syncytial virus (RSV). Wait times in ERs in children's hospitals have climbed up to shockingly high numbers. In my home province, a precious five-year-old girl from Northern British Columbia died from influenza after being taken to a city hospital. A few days later, the premier and the provincial health officer appeared grinning and maskless at a packed hospital fundraising gala. This is a sickening "let them eat cake" moment in Canada, where the rich congratulate themselves while babies are dying.

This new revolution will not be born out of Canadian politeness. Fight as hard as you can for equitable healthcare for all before it's too late.

My friend, environmentalist and social justice activist Mary Morgan, died in April 2021. During our last phone conversation, she told me to keep fighting, but to also pause and find joy too. Seek out joy in the midst of this darkness, dear readers, for hope lives in that joy.

Now roll up your sleeves. We have work to do.

SUE ROBINS is a healthcare activist, speaker, and author. Her latest book, *Ducks in a Row: Health Care Reimagined*, is a scrappy challenge to the established healthcare world. She is also the senior partner in the creative health communications company Bird Comm. Sue has written for the *New York Times*, *Canadian Medical Association Journal*, and the *Globe and Mail*.

Notes

Introduction: I Can't. I'm Too Broken

1 Government of Canada, "COVID-19 Epidemiology Update: Summary," last updated 23 September 2022, https://health-infobase.canada.ca.

2 Nili Kaplan-Myrth, "Be Afraid of COVID-19: I Am," *Ottawa Citizen*, 6 October 2020, https://ottawacitizen.com/opinion/dr-nili-kaplan-myrth -be-afraid-of-covid-19-i-am.

3 Ontario COVID-19 Science Advisory Table, "Update on COVID-19 Projections: Science Advisory and Modelling Consensus Tables," 1 September 2021, https://covid19-sciencetable.ca/wp-content/uploads/2021/09 /Update-on-COVID-19-Projections_2021.09.01_English-1.pdf.

4 Centers for Disease Control and Prevention, "Global Orphanhood Associated with COVID-19," last updated 25 October 2022, https://www.cdc. gov/globalhealth/covid-19/orphanhood/index.html#:~:text=The%20 number%20of%20children%20who,co%2Dled%20by%20CDC%20reveals.

Chapter 4: A Community Divided

1 For example, the United Church and the Baptist Church provided online services to protect their members. Eddie Rempel, executive director of Mennonite Community Services, stated that his organization provided regular updates from public health on a local German radio station to support newcomers. See Isha Bhargava, "Postal Code N5H in Aylmer, Ont., Has Lowest Vaccination Rate in the Province," *CBC News*, last updated 11 November 2021, https://www.cbc.ca/news/canada/london/postal-code -n5h-in-aylmer-ont-has-lowest-vaccination-rate-in-the-province-1.6244416.

2 Jane Sims, "Aylmer's Church of God Loses COVID-19 Court Challenge," *London Free Press*, 2 March 2022, https://lfpress.com/news/local-news /aylmers-church-of-god-loses-covid-19-court-challenge.
3 The CTV program *W5* produced a documentary on coercive control over COGR's members: "W5: Controversial Religious Sect in Small-Town Ontario Preaches Disruption," YouTube, 22:39, 22 October 2019, https:// www.youtube.com/watch?v=dNskfQpjsag.

Chapter 5: BC – Breaking Cancer

1 Bridgette Watson and Deborah Wilson, "In 1991, B.C. Had More Family Doctors than It Needed. So Why Are So Many Residents Unable to Find One Now?," *CBC News*, 28 April 2022, https://www.cbc.ca/news /canada/british-columbia/bc-health-care-history-1.6431301.
2 PoP BC, "The Missing Voices: Stories from the Front Lines of BC Hospitals," 17 November 2021, https://protectbc.ca/stories-from-bcs-hospital -front-lines-the-missing-voices/.

Chapter 6: Learning to Count

1 "Cumulative Confirmed COVID-19 Deaths," Our World in Data, accessed 31 May 2023, https://ourworldindata.org/explorers/coronavirus -data-explorer?facet=none&Metric=Confirmed+deaths&Interval =Cumulative&Relative+to+Population=false&Color+by+test+positivity =false&country=~CAN.
2 G. Douaud et al., "SARS-CoV-2 Is Associated with Changes in Brain Structure in UK Biobank," *Nature* 604 (2022): 697–707, https://www .nature.com/articles/s41586-022-04569-5; Ioannis Katsoularis, "Risks of Deep Vein Thrombosis, Pulmonary Embolism, and Bleeding after COVID-19: Nationwide Self-Controlled Cases Series and Matched Cohort Study," *BMJ* 377 (2022): e069590, https://www.bmj.com/content/377 /bmj-2021-069590; and Panagis Galiatsatos, "COVID-19 Lung Damage," Johns Hopkins Medicine, last updated 28 February 2022, https://www .hopkinsmedicine.org/health/conditions-and-diseases/coronavirus /what-coronavirus-does-to-the-lungs.

Chapter 7: The Spring

1 Ontario Ministry of Health, Ministry of Long-Term Care, "Severe Acute Respiratory Syndrome (SARS)," last updated 8 August 2018, https:// web.archive.org/web/20220325185948/http://www.health.gov.on.ca:80 /en/public/publications/pub_sars.aspx.
2 Alex Boyd, "Jason Kenney Lays Out Plan for 'The Best Alberta Summer Ever' – with COVID Reopening That Outpaces Ontario," *Toronto Star*, 26 May 2021, https://www.thestar.com/news/canada/2021/05/26 /weeks-after-facing-north-americas-highest-covid-rates-alberta-unveils -plan-to-almost-fully-reopen-by-early-july.html.

3 Trisha Greenhalgh et al., "Ten Scientific Reasons in Support of Airborne Transmission of SARS-CoV-2," *The Lancet* 397, no. 10285 (2021): 1603–5, https://doi.org/10.1016/S0140-6736(21)00869-2.
4 Anuradhaa Subramanian et al., "Symptoms and Risk Factors for Long COVID in Non-hospitalized Adults," *Nature Medicine* 28, no. 8 (2022): 1706–14, https://doi.org/10.1038/s41591-022-01909-w.
5 Ziyad Al-Aly, Benjamin Bowe, and Yan Xie, "Outcomes of SARS-CoV-2 Reinfection" (Preprint, submitted 17 June 2022), https://doi.org/10.21203/rs.3.rs-1749502/v1.
6 Public Health Agency of Canada, "Post COVID-19 Condition (Long COVID)," last updated 9 March 2023, https://www.canada.ca/en/public-health/services/diseases/2019-novel-coronavirus-infection/symptoms/post-covid-19-condition.html.
7 Ziyad Al-Aly, Yan Xie, and Benjamin Bowe, "High-Dimensional Characterization of Post-Acute Sequelae of COVID-19," *Nature* 594 (2021): 259–64, https://doi.org/10.1038/s41586-021-03553-9.

Chapter 8: Long-Term Care or Long-Term Crime?

1 Rona Ambrose, "Seniors' Care-Home Neglect Is Our National Shame," *Globe and Mail*, 13 April 2020, https://www.theglobeandmail.com/opinion/article-seniors-care-home-neglect-is-our-national-shame/.
2 Canadian Institute for Health Information, *Pandemic Experience in the Long-Term Care Sector: How Does Canada Compare with Other Countries?* (Ottawa: CIHI, 2020), https://www.cihi.ca/sites/default/files/document/covid-19-rapid-response-long-term-care-snapshot-en.pdf.
3 Murray Brewster and Vassy Kapelos, "Military Alleges Horrific Conditions, Abuse in Pandemic-Hit Ontario Nursing Homes," *CBC News*, last updated 27 May 2020, https://www.cbc.ca/news/politics/long-term-care-pandemic-covid-coronavirus-trudeau-1.5584960.
4 Emilio Parodi, "Uncounted among Coronavirus Victims, Deaths Sweep through Italy's Nursing Homes," Reuters, 18 March 2020, https://www.reuters.com/article/us-health-coronavirus-italy-homes-insigh-idUSKBN2152V0.
5 Marco Trabucchi and Diego de Leo, "Nursing Homes or Abandoned Castles: COVID-19 in Italy," *The Lancet Psychiatry* 8, no. 2 (2021): e6, https://www.thelancet.com/journals/lanpsy/article/PIIS2215-0366(20)30541-1/fulltext.
6 Trabucchi and Leo, "Nursing Homes or Abandoned Castles."
7 Sara Berloto, Elisabetta Notarnicola, Eleonora Perobelli, and Andrea Rotolo, "Report on COVID-19 and Long-Term Care in Italy: Lessons Learned from an Absent Crisis Management," LTC Responses to COVID-19, 10 April 2020, https://ltccovid.org/2020/04/10/report-on-covid-19-and-long-term-care-in-italy-lessons-learned-from-an-absent-crisis-management/; Flavia Lombardo et al., "Adverse Events in Italian Nursing Homes during the COVID-19 Epidemic: A

National Survey," *Frontiers in Psychiatry* 11 (2020): 578465, https://doi
.org/10.3389/fpsyt.2020.578465.

8 Greta Privitera, "The 'Silent Massacre' in Italy's Nursing Homes: Care
Homes for the Elderly Have Become Hotbeds of the Coronavirus Epidemic,"
POLITICO, 30 April 2020, https://www.politico.eu/article/the-silent
-coronavirus-covid19-massacre-in-italy-milan-lombardy-nursing-care
-homes-elderly/.

9 Louise E. Lansbury, Caroline S. Brown, and Jonathan S. Nguyen-Van
-Tam, "Influenza in Long-Term Care Facilities," *Influenza and Other Respiratory Viruses* 11, no. 5 (2017): 356–66, https://www.ncbi.nlm.nih.gov
/pmc/articles/PMC5596516/.

10 Michael Liu et al., "COVID-19 in Long-Term Care Homes in Ontario and
British Columbia," *CMAJ* 192, no. 47 (2020): e1540–6, https://www.cmaj
.ca/content/192/47/E1540.

11 Mike Hager and Andrea Woo, "How the Coronavirus Took North Vancouver's Lynn Valley Care Centre," *Globe and Mail*, 21 March 2020, https://
www.theglobeandmail.com/canada/article-how-the-coronavirus
-took-north-vancouvers-lynn-valley-care-centre/.

12 Adam Carter, "Ontario's Long-Term Care Sector Wasn't Ready or Equipped
for COVID-19: Report," *CBC News*, last updated 29 April 2021, https://www
.cbc.ca/news/canada/toronto/long-term-care-pandemic-report-1.6005331.

13 Charlene Harrington et al., "Nursing Home Staffing Standards and Staffing Levels in Six Countries," *Journal of Nursing Scholarship* 44, no. 1 (2012):
88–98, https://pubmed.ncbi.nlm.nih.gov/22340814/.

14 Charlene H. Chu, Simon Donato-Woodger, and Christopher J. Dainton,
"Competing Crises: COVID-19 Countermeasures and Social Isolation
among Older Adults in Long-Term Care," *Journal of Advanced Nursing*
76, no. 10 (2020): 2456–9, https://www.ncbi.nlm.nih.gov/pmc/articles/
PMC7361866/.

15 Vivian Stamatopoulos, "Not Just a Visitor: It's Time to Allow Essential
Family Caregivers Back into Long-Term Care Homes," Ontario Tech University, 5 May 2020, https://socialscienceandhumanities.ontariotechu.ca
/about/faculty-blog/archives/not-just-a-visitor-its-time-to-allow-essential
-family-caregivers-back-into-long-term-care-homes.php; Vivian Stamatopoulos, "What Happened to Residents' Rights? How Blanket Family
Bans Violate Ontario's Long-Term Care Homes Act," Ontario Tech University, 11 May 2020, https://socialscienceandhumanities.ontariotechu.ca
/about/faculty-blog/archives/what-happened-to-residents-rights-how
-blanket-family-bans-violate-ontarios-long-term-care-homes-act.php;
Vivian Stamatopoulos, "Missing the Mark: Ontario's Ongoing Refusal
to Recognize Family Caregivers as 'Essential,'" DurhamRegion.com, 24
July 2020, https://www.durhamregion.com/opinion-story/10111766
-missing-the-mark-ontario-s-ongoing-refusal-to-recognize-family
-caregivers-as-essential-/; Vivian Stamatopoulos, "Who Is Going to
Protect Our Seniors in Long-Term Care?," DurhamRegion.com, 3
June 2020, https://www.durhamregion.com/opinion/who-is-going-to

-protect-our-seniors-in-long-term-care/article_48c032c7-0588-597b-852d
-16235dbfb614.html.

16 Anna Nienhuis, "Uniting Government across Party Lines to Reform
LTC," *Hamilton Spectator*, 12 February 2021, https://www.thespec.com
/opinion/contributors/2021/02/12/uniting-government-across-party
-lines-to-reform-ltc.html.

17 Amit Arya, Amina Jabbar, and Vivian Stamatopoulos, "Preparing Nursing Homes for a Second Wave Starts with Staffing," *Toronto Star*, 27
August 2020, https://www.thestar.com/opinion/contributors/2020/08
/27/preparing-nursing-homes-for-a-second-wave-starts-with-staffing
.html; Jennifer Yang and Sara Mojtehedzadeh, "Ontario Let a 'Flood' of
Temp Agencies into Long-Term Care during COVID-19. How Precarious
Work Put Residents and Caregivers at Risk," *Toronto Star*, 18 March 2021,
https://www.thestar.com/news/gta/2021/03/18/ontario-let-a-flood-of
-temp-agencies-into-long-term-care-during-COVID-19-how-precarious
-work-put-residents-and-caregivers-at-risk.html; and Jennifer Yang,
"He Disinfected Subways, Helped Disabled Adults and Worked as a
PSW during a COVID-19 Outbreak. What One Temp Worker Wants
You to Know about Life on the Pandemic Front Lines," *Toronto Star*,
20 March 2021, https://www.thestar.com/news/gta/2021/03/20/he
-disinfected-subways-helped-disabled-adults-and-worked-as-a-psw
-during-a-COVID-19-outbreak-what-one-temp-worker-wants-you-to
-know-about-life-on-the-pandemic-front-lines.html.

18 Rosie DiManno, "The Military's Report Details the Horrors of Ontario
Long-Term-Care Homes. Shame on All of Us for Letting It Happen,"
Toronto Star, 26 May 2020, https://www.thestar.com/opinion/star
-columnists/2020/05/26/the-militarys-report-details-the-horrors-of
-long-term-care-homes-shame-on-all-of-us-for-letting-it-happen.html.

19 4th Canadian Division Joint Task Force, "Observations in Long-Term
Care Facilities in Ontario," May 2020, https://www.macleans.ca/wp
-content/uploads/2020/05/JTFC-Observations-in-LTCF-in-ON.pdf.

20 Nili Kaplan-Myrth and Amy Tan, "Reflections on a Pan-Canadian
Round Table on COVID-19 Vaccination," *CMAJ Blogs*, 8 March 2021,
https://cmajblogs.com/reflections-on-a-pan-canadian-round-table
-on-covid-19-vaccination/; Canadians4LTC, "Expert Roundtable with
Prime Minister Justin Trudeau," YouTube, https://www.youtube.com
/watch?v=PvuB4iJ7Ab4; CPAC, "PM Trudeau Holds Roundtable with
Health-Care Workers – February 11, 2021," YouTube, https://www
.youtube.com/watch?v=rqjYP7dimhQ.

21 Charlene H. Chu, Amanda V. Yee, and Vivian Stamatopoulos, "'It's the
Worst Thing I've Ever Been Put Through in My Life': The Trauma Experienced by Essential Family Caregivers of Loved Ones in Long-Term Care
during the COVID-19 Pandemic In Canada," *International Journal of Qualitative Studies on Health and Well-Being* 17, no. 1 (2022): 2075532, https://
doi.org/10.1080/17482631.2022.2075532; Charlene H. Chu and Vivian Stamatopoulos, "Caregivers Were Traumatized by COVID-19 Public Health

and Long-Term Care Policies," *The Conversation*, 17 July 2022, https://theconversation.com/caregivers-were-traumatized-by-covid-19-public-health-and-long-term-care-policies-185109; Charlene H. Chu, Amanda Yee, and Vivian Stamatopoulos, "Poor and Lost Connections: Essential Family Caregivers' Experiences Using Technology with Family Living in Long-Term Care Homes during COVID-19," *Journal of Applied Gerontology* 41, no. 6 (2022): 1547–56, https://doi.org/10.1177/07334648221081850; and Toronto Star Editorial Board, "Open Doors to Family Caregivers," *Toronto Star*, 18 July 2022, https://www.thestar.com/opinion/editorials/2022/07/18/open-doors-to-family-caregivers.html.

22 National Institute on Ageing, *Counting COVID-19 in Canada's Long-Term Care Homes: NIA Long-Term Care COVID-19 Tracker Project Summary Report* (Toronto: National Institute on Ageing and Toronto Metropolitan University, 2022), https://static1.squarespace.com/static/5c2fa7b03917eed9b5a436d8/t/62e20cf7815ce31282864f3a/1658981624185/NIA_LTCtracker_V6+-Final.pdf.

23 The Canadian Press, "Non-Profit Long-Term Care Homes Have Lost Too Many Residents to COVID-19," *National Post*, 9 June 2021, https://nationalpost.com/pmn/news-pmn/non-profit-long-term-care-homes-have-lost-too-many-residents-to-covid-19.

24 CBC Radio, "Canada's For-Profit Model of Long-Term Care Has Failed the Elderly, Says Leading Expert," *The Sunday Magazine*, 24 April 2020, https://www.cbc.ca/radio/sunday/the-sunday-edition-for-april-26-2020-1.5536429/canada-s-for-profit-model-of-long-term-care-has-failed-the-elderly-says-leading-expert-1.5540891; and Pat Armstrong and Hugh Armstrong, eds., *The Privatization of Care: The Case of Nursing Homes* (New York: Routledge, 2019).

25 Nathan M. Stall et al., "COVID-19 and Ontario's Long-Term Care Homes," *Science Briefs of the Ontario COVID-19 Science Advisory Table*, 1, no. 7 (2021), https://doi.org/10.47326/ocsat.2021.02.07.1.0, https://covid19-sciencetable.ca/wp-content/uploads/2021/01/Science-Brief_Full-Brief_COVID-19-and-Ontarios-Long-Term-Care-Homes_published-1.pdf.

26 Ed Tubb, Kenyon Wallace, and Brendan Kennedy, "For-Profit Nursing Homes in Ontario Say Ownership Has Nothing to Do with Their Higher COVID-19 Death Rates. A Star Analysis Finds That's Not the Case," *Toronto Star*, 26 February 2021, https://www.thestar.com/business/2021/02/26/for-profit-nursing-homes-say-ownership-has-nothing-to-do-with-their-higher-covid-19-death-rates-a-star-analysis-finds-thats-not-the-case.html.

27 Kenyon Wallace, Ed Tubb, and Marco Chown Oved, "Big For-Profit Long-Term-Care Companies Paid Out More than $170 Million to Investors through Ontario's Deadly First Wave," *Toronto Star*, 26 December 2020, https://www.thestar.com/news/gta/2020/12/26/big-for-profit-long-term-care-companies-paid-out-more-than-170-million-to-investors-through-ontarios-deadly-first-wave.html.

28 "Long-Term Care COVID-19 Commission Meeting, Dr. David Williams, Chief Medical Officer of Health, on Monday, February 22, 2021"

(Toronto: Neesons Reporting, 2021), https://wayback.archive-it.
org/17275/20210810151125/http://www.ltccommission-commission-
sld.ca/transcripts/pdf/Dr._David_Williams_Chief_Medical_Officer_of
_Health_Transcript_February_22_2021.pdf.
29 Frank N. Marrocco, Angela Coke, and Dr. Jack Kitts, *Ontario's Long-Term Care COVID-19 Commission: Final Report* (Toronto: Queen's Printer for Ontario, 2021), https://www.ontario.ca/page/long-term-care-covid-19
-commission-progress-interim-recommendations.
30 Vivian Stamatopoulos and Natalie Mehra, "Keeping Private Long-Term Care Would Be a Deadly Mistake," *Toronto Star*, 10 February 2021, https://www.thestar.com/opinion/contributors/keeping-private-long-term-care-would-be-a-deadly-mistake/article_1e4569b6-1010-5bd7
-bcb3-cc77ed7e0f2e.html.
31 Marco Chown Oved, Kenyon Wallace, and Ed Tubb, "Doug Ford Is Spending Billions to Expand Nursing Home Chains with Some of the Worst COVID-19 Death Rates," *Toronto Star*, 27 May 2022, https://www
.thestar.com/news/investigations/2022/05/27/doug-ford-is-spending
-billions-to-expand-nursing-home-chains-with-some-of-the-worst-covid
-19-death-rates.html.
32 Brendan Ellis, "SHA to Assume Operation of Sask. Extendicare Long
-Term Care Homes," *CTV News Regina*, 14 October 2021,https://regina
.ctvnews.ca/sha-to-assume-operation-of-sask-extendicare-long-term
-care-homes-1.5623036.
33 Bruce Campion-Smith, "Canadians Favour Overhaul of Long-Term-Care Homes, Survey Shows," *Toronto Star*, 26 May 2020, https://www.thestar
.com/politics/federal/2020/05/26/canadians-favour-overhaul-of-long
-term-care-homes-survey-shows.html.
34 Inori Roy and Tai Huynh, "Who's Actually Running Ontario's Long
-Term Care Homes?," The Local, 15 January 2021, https://thelocal.to
/whos-actually-running-ontarios-long-term-care-homes/.
35 Erin Fleury and Heather Campbell, "Recent Legal Developments: Video Surveillance in Care Homes," Canadian Network for the Prevention of Elder Abuse, 18 January 2016, https://cnpea.ca/en/about-cnpea
/blog/520-recent-legal-developments-video-surveillance-in-care
-homes.
36 "Long-Term Care in Ontario," Government of Ontario, last updated 24 March 2023, https://www.ontario.ca/page/long-term-care-ontario.
37 Victoria Gibson, "More Than 1/3 of Ontario LTC Facilities Report Increases in Worsening Pressure Ulcers, Chemical or Physical Restraint Use," *iPolitics*, 2 June 2020, https://ipolitics.ca/news/more-than-1-3
-of-ontario-ltc-facilities-report-increases-in-worsening-pressure
-ulcers-chemical-or-physical-restraint-use.
38 Elizabeth Payne, "'Unfair and Inhumane': MPPs Pass Voula's Law to Prevent Families Being Kept Out of Care Homes," *Ottawa Citizen*, 8 March 2021, https://ottawacitizen.com/news/local-news/unfair-and
-inhumane-mpps-pass-voulas-law-to-prevent-families-being-kept-out
-of-care-homes.

Chapter 9: Go Home

1 Jing Hui Wang and Greg Moreau, "Police-Reported Hate Crime in Canada," Statistics Canada, 17 March 2022, https://www150.statcan .gc.ca/n1/pub/85-002-x/2022001/article/00005-eng.htm.

Chapter 10: Ableism

1 Statistics Canada, "Low Income Cut-Offs (LICOs) before and after Tax by Community Size and Family Size, in Current Dollars," 2 May 2023, https://www150.statcan.gc.ca/t1/tbl1/en/tv.action?pid=1110024101.
2 Income Security Advocacy Centre, "OW & ODSP Rates and the Ontario Child Benefit – Current to September 2022," accessed 1 June 2023, https://incomesecurity.org/wp-content/uploads/2022/09/Sept-2022 -OW-and-ODSP-rates-and-OCB-EN.pdf.

Chapter 12: The Pandemic Changed Nothing

1 "The Honourable Carla Qualtrough," Government of Canada, accessed 5 June 2023, https://pm.gc.ca/en/cabinet/honourable-carla-qualtrough.
2 "One-Time Payment to Persons with Disabilities," Government of Canada, accessed 5 June 2023, https://www.canada.ca/en/services/benefits /one-time-payment-persons-disabilities.html.
3 Jennefer Laidley and Mohy Tabbara, *Welfare in Canada, 2020* (Toronto: Maytree, 2021), https://maytree.com/wp-content/uploads/Welfare_in _Canada_2020.pdf.
4 Stuart Morris, Gail Fawcett, Laurent Brisebois, and Jeffrey Hughes, "Canadian Survey on Disability Reports: A Demographic, Employment and Income Profile of Canadians with Disabilities Aged 15 Years and Over, 2017," Statistics Canada, 28 November 2018, https://www150.statcan .gc.ca/n1/pub/89-654-x/89-654-x2018002-eng.htm.
5 "Medical Assistance in Dying," Government of Canada, last updated 1 June 2023, https://www.canada.ca/en/health-canada/services/medical -assistance-dying.html.
6 Health Canada, *Third Annual Report on MAID in Canada 2021* (Ottawa: Government of Canada, 2022), https://www.canada.ca/en/health -canada/services/medical-assistance-dying/annual-report-2021.html.

Chapter 13: Wild Teens

1 Aristotle, *Rhetoric*, trans. W. Rhys Roberts (North Chelmsford, MA: Courier, 2004), book II, chap. 12.
2 Erik H. Erikson, *Identity, Youth, and Crisis* (New York: W.W. Norton, 1968).
3 Studies in functional magnetic resonance imaging (fMRI) have demonstrated variability between adults' and adolescents' brains when making

decisions. Valerie Reyna and Frank Farley, "Risk and Rationality in Adolescent Decision Making: Implications for Theory, Practice and Public Policy," *Psychological Science in the Public Interest* 7, no. 1 (2006): 1–44, https://doi.org/10.1111/j.1529-1006.2006.00026.x.

4 Ying Sun et al., "Comparison of Mental Health Symptoms before and during the Covid-19 Pandemic: Evidence from a Systematic Review and Meta-Analysis of 134 Cohorts," *BMJ Clinical Research* 380 (2023): e074224, https://www.bmj.com/content/380/bmj-2022-074224.

Chapter 15: Resilience Is a Dirty Word

1 Registered Nurses' Association of Ontario, "Ontario's RN Understaffing Crisis: Impact and Solution," Political Action Bulletin, November 2022, https://rnao.ca/sites/default/files/2021-11/Ontarios%20RN%20understaffing%20Crisis%20Impact%20and%20Solution%20PAB%202021.pdf.

2 Canadian Federation of Nurses Unions, "New Study Reveals Shocking Levels of Mental Illness among Canada's Nurses," Media Release, 16 June 2020, https://nursesunions.ca/new-study-reveals-shocking-levels-of-mental-illness-among-canadas-nurses/.

3 Canadian Federation of Nurses Unions, "Canada's Nursing Shortage at a Glance: A Media Reference Guide," January 2022, https://nursesunions.ca/wp-content/uploads/2022/07/nurses_shortage_media_ref_guide_comp.pdf.

4 David Barrett and Alison Twycross, "Impact of COVID-19 on Nursing Students' Mental Health: A Systematic Review and Meta-Analysis," *Evidence-Based Nursing* 25, no. 1 (2022): 8–9, https://doi.org/10.1136/ebnurs-2021-103500.

5 Statistics Canada, "Experiences of Health Care Workers during the COVID-19 Pandemic, September to November 2021," The Daily, 3 June 2022, https://www150.statcan.gc.ca/n1/daily-quotidien/220603/dq220603a-eng.htm.

6 Pete Evans, "Canada Lost 31,000 Jobs Last Month, the Second Straight Monthly Decline," *CBC News*, 5 August 2022, https://www.cbc.ca/news/business/canada-jobs-july-1.6542271.

7 Muriel Draaisma, "Physical Violence 'Part of the Job' for Hospital Workers, CUPE Poll Finds," *CBC News*, 5 July 2022, https://www.cbc.ca/news/canada/toronto/cupe-poll-hospital-workers-ontario-violence-1.6511265.

8 Andrea M. Stelnicki, R. Nicholas Carleton, and Carol Reichert, *Mental Disorder Symptoms among Nurses in Canada* (Ottawa: Canadian Federation of Nurses Unions, 2020), https://nursesunions.ca/research/mental-disorder-symptoms/.

9 Ontario Nurses Association, "Ontario's Nurse Staffing Is Falling Further behind the Rest of Canada," News Release, 17 November 2022, https://www.ona.org/news-posts/20221117-nurse-staffing-report/.

10 Ontario Nurses Association, "Ontario's Nurse Staffing."

11 Houssem Edine Ben Ahmed and Ivy Lynn Bourgeault, *Sustaining Nursing in Canada: A Set of Coordinated Evidence-Based Solutions Targeted to Support the Nursing Workforce Now and into the Future* (Ottawa: Canadian Federation of Nurses Unions, 2022), https://nursesunions.ca/research/sustaining-nursing-in-canada-a-set-of-coordinated-evidence-based-solutions-targeted-to-support-the-nursing-workforce-now-and-into-the-future/.

Chapter 16: Men Write the Policies, Women Face the Results

1 Anonymous, "The Punishment of Being a Nurse," 14 August 2022, mycovidstory.ca (site discontinued).
2 World Health Organization, *Delivered by Women, Led by Men: A Gender and Equity Analysis of the Global Health and Social Workforce* (Geneva: WHO, 2019), https://apps.who.int/iris/handle/10665/311322.
3 The full title of the employment category "health and social workforce" has been shortened in this essay to "health workforce" for readability.
4 The Sex, Gender and Covid-19 Project, "Sex-Disaggregated Data Tracker," last updated 15 September 2022, https://globalhealth5050.org/the-sex-gender-and-covid-19-project/the-data-tracker/?explore=country&country=Canada#search.
5 Statistics Canada, "Employment by Class of Worker, Annual," 6 January 2023, https://www150.statcan.gc.ca/t1/tbl1/en/tv.action?pid=1410002701.
6 Wendy Glauser, "Rise of Women in Medicine Not Matched by Leadership Roles," *Canadian Medical Association Journal* 190, no. 15 (2018): e479–80, https://doi.org/10.1503/cmaj.109-5567.
7 Lokpriy Sharma and Julia Smith, "Women in a COVID-19 Recession: Employment, Job Loss and Wage Inequality in Canada," Gender and Covid-19 Evidence Download, 2021, https://www.genderandcovid-19.org/wp-content/uploads/2021/06/Women-in-a-COVID-19-recession-Canada-and-economic-impacts.pdf; and Janet Lum, Jennifer Sladek, and Alvin Ying, *Ontario Personal Support Workers in Home and Community Care: CRNCC/PSNO Survey Results* (Toronto: Ryerson University, 2010), https://www.torontomu.ca/content/dam/crncc/knowledge/infocus/factsheets/InFocus-Ontario%20PSWs%20in%20Home%20and%20Community%20Care.pdf.
8 BC Women's Health Foundation, *Invisible No More* (29 November 2021), 8, https://assets.bcwomensfoundation.org/2021/11/29160837/BCWHF-invisiblenomore-report-full-FINAL-Nov29.pdf.
9 Marilou Gagnon et al., "Blowing the Whistle during the First Wave of COVID-19: A Case Study of Quebec Nurses," *Journal of Advanced Nursing* 78, no. 12 (2022): 1–15, https://doi.org/10.1111/jan.15365.
10 The Sex, Gender and Covid-19 Project, "Sex-Disaggregated Data Tracker."
11 Canadian Institute for Health Information, "COVID-19 Cases and Deaths in Health Care Workers in Canada – Data Tables," 31 March 2022, https://www.cihi.ca/en/covid-19-cases-and-deaths-in-health-care-workers-in-canada.

12 Canadian Institute for Health Information, *The Impact of COVID-19 on Long-Term Care in Canada: Focus on the First 6 Months* (Ottawa: CIHI, 2021), https://www.cihi.ca/sites/default/files/document/impact-covid-19 -long-term-care-canada-first-6-months-report-en.pdf.

13 Carole A. Estabrooks and Janice Keefe, "COVID-19 Crisis in Nursing Homes Is a Gender Crisis," *Policy Options*, 19 May 2020, https:// policyoptions.irpp.org/magazines/may-2020/covid-19-crisis-in -nursing-homes-is-a-gender-crisis/.

14 The Sex, Gender and Covid-19 Project, "Sex-Disaggregated Data Tracker."

15 Les Perreaux, "Women Make Up over Half of COVID-19 Deaths in Canada, Counter to Trends in Most of World," *Globe and Mail*, 20 May 2020, https://www.theglobeandmail.com/canada/article-women-make-up -over-half-of-covid-19-deaths-in-canada-counter-to/.

16 The Sex, Gender and Covid-19 Project, "Sex-Disaggregated Data Tracker."

17 Public Health Agency of Canada, "Infections among Healthcare Workers and Other People Working in Healthcare Settings," Government of Canada, last updated 4 March 2022, https://www.canada.ca/en /public-health/services/diseases/coronavirus-disease-covid-19 /epidemiological-economic-research-data/infections-healthcare -workers-other-people-working-healthcare-settings.html.

18 The Sex, Gender and Covid-19 Project, "Sex-Disaggregated Data Tracker."

19 Niki Oveisi et al., *The Experiences of Nurses in British Columbia, Canada during COVID-19* (Vancouver: Gender & COVID-19 Project, 2021), 1, https://www.genderandcovid-19.org/wp-content/uploads/2021/10 /PAC00475_Gender-and-Covid-19-Nurses-Brief-BCWHF.pdf.

20 Tina James, "'Two Weeks After I Started My Job in Long-Term Care, I Tested Positive': A PSW Tells Her Story," *Toronto Life*, 18 January 2021, https://torontolife.com/city/two-weeks-after-i-started-my-job-in-long -term-care-i-tested-positive-a-psw-tells-her-story/.

21 James, "Two Weeks After."

22 James, "Two Weeks After."

23 Ontario Ministry of Long-Term Care, *Long-Term Care Staffing Study* (Toronto: Ministry of Long Term Care, 2020), 8, https://www.ontario.ca /page/long-term-care-staffing-study.

24 Katherine Zagrodney and Mike Saks, "Personal Support Workers in Canada: The New Precariat?," *Healthcare Policy* 13, no. 2 (2017): 31–9, https://www.longwoods.com/content/25324/healthcare-policy /personal-support-workers-in-canada-the-new-precariat-.

25 Canadian Institute for Health Information, "The Impact of COVID-19 on Canada's Long-Term Care Workers," 17 November 2022, https:// www.cihi.ca/en/health-workforce-in-canada-highlights-of-the-impact -of-covid-19/the-impact-of-covid-19-on-canadas; and Ayu Pinky Hapsari et al., "The Working Conditions for Personal Support Workers in the Greater Toronto Area during the COVID-19 Pandemic: A Mixed-Methods Study," *Canadian Journal of Public Health* 113, no. 6 (2022): 817–33, https:// doi.org/10.17269/s41997-022-00643-7.

26 Gender & Covid-19, "'We're Just Treated So Differently': Experiences of Women Working in Long-Term Care Facilities in British Columbia, Canada during COVID-19" (Vancouver: Gender & Covid-19, 2021), 1, https://www.genderandcovid-19.org/wp-content/uploads/2021/12 /Women-working-in-long-term-care-facilities-in-British-Columbia.pdf.

27 CBC Radio, "PSW Draws Attention to 'Burnt Out' Staff as COVID-19 Compounds Long-Term Care Crisis," *White Coat, Black Art*, 8 May 2020, https://www.cbc.ca/radio/whitecoat/psw-draws-attention-to-burnt -out-staff-as-covid-19-compounds-long-term-care-crisis-1.5556752.

28 Lum, Sladek, and Ying, *Ontario Personal Support Workers*.

29 Martin Turcotte and Katherine Savage, *The Contribution of Immigrants and Population Groups Designated as Visible Minorities to Nurse Aide, Orderly and Patient Service Associate Occupations* (Ottawa: Statistics Canada, 2020), 4, https://www150.statcan.gc.ca/n1/pub/45-28-0001/2020001 /article/00036-eng.htm.

30 Louis Cornelissen, *Profile of Immigrants in Nursing and Health Care Support Occupations* (Ottawa: Statistics Canada, 2021), https://www150.statcan .gc.ca/n1/pub/75-006-x/2021001/article/00004-eng.htm.

31 A. Pinto et al., "Precarious Work among Personal Support Workers in the Greater Toronto Area: A Respondent-Driven Sampling Study," *CMAJO* 10, no. 2 (2022): e527–38, https://doi.org/10.9778/cmajo.20210338.

32 Lena Gahwi and Margaret Walton-Roberts, "Migrant Care Labour, Covid-19, and the Long-Term Care Crisis: Achieving Solidarity for Care Providers and Recipients," in *Migration and Pandemics: Spaces of Solidarity and Spaces of Exception*, ed. Anna Triandafyllidou, IMISCOE Research Series (Cham: Springer, 2021), 108, https://link.springer.com /chapter/10.1007/978-3-030-81210-2_6.

33 Carieta Thomas and Naomi Lightman, "'Island Girls': Caribbean Women Care Workers in Canada," *Canadian Ethnic Studies* 54, no. 1 (2022): 29–58, https://doi.org/10.1353/ces.2022.0004.

34 Rajendra Subedi, Lawson Greenberg, and Martin Turcotte, *COVID-19 Mortality Rates in Canada's Ethno-Cultural Neighbourhoods* (Ottawa: Statistics Canada, 2020), 3, https://www150.statcan.gc.ca/n1/pub/45-28 -0001/2020001/article/00079-eng.pdf.

35 BC Women's Health Foundation, *Invisible No More*.

36 Julia Smith et al., "'I May Be Essential but Someone Has to Look after My Kids': Women Physicians and Covid-19," *Canadian Journal of Public Health* 113, no. 1 (2022): 107–16, https://doi.org/10.17269/s41997-021-00595-4.

37 Sharma and Smith, "Women in a COVID-19 Recession."

38 Smith et al., "I May Be Essential."

39 Lael M. Yonker et al., "Virologic Features of Severe Acute Respiratory Syndrome Coronavirus 2 Infection in Children," *The Journal of Infectious Diseases* 224, no. 11 (2021): 1821–9, https://doi.org/10.1093/infdis/jiab509.

40 Julia Smith et al., "More Than a Public Health Crisis: A Feminist Political Economic Analysis of COVID-19," *Global Public Health* 16, no. 8–9 (2021): 1364–80, https://doi.org/10.1080/17441692.2021.1896765.

41 Smith et al., "I May Be Essential."
42 Trevor van Ingen et al., "Neighbourhood-Level Risk Factors of COVID-19 Incidence and Mortality," *medRxiv* (preprint, submitted 1 January 2021), https://doi.org/10.1101/2021.01.27.21250618.
43 Smith et al., "I May Be Essential."
44 Oveisi et al., "The Experiences of Nurses in British Columbia," 6.
45 Fatemeh Torabi Asr et al., "The Gender Gap Tracker: Using Natural Language Processing to Measure Gender Bias in Media," *PLOS ONE* 16, no. 1 (2021): e0245533, https://doi.org/10.1371/journal.pone.0245533.
46 Maite Taboada, "The Coronavirus Pandemic Increased the Visibility of Women in the Media, but It's Not All Good News," *The Conversation*, 25 November 2020, https://theconversation.com/the-coronavirus -pandemic-increased-the-visibility-of-women-in-the-media-but-its-not -all-good-news-146389.
47 Prashanth Rao, Lucas Chambers, and Maite Taboada, "Three Years of Monitoring Gender Representation in the Media," SFU, Discourse Processing Lab, 7 July 2022, https://www.sfu.ca/discourse-lab/research /GGT-3years.html.
48 Diana J. Mason et al., "The Woodhull Study Revisited: Nurses' Representation in Health News Media 20 Years Later," *Journal of Nursing Scholarship* 50, no. 6 (2018): 695–704, https://doi.org/10.1111/jnu.12429.
49 While only 22 per cent of adult intensivists are female, the proportion of female pediatric intensivists is higher at 52 per cent. See Canadian Institute for Health Information, "Physicians," accessed 6 July 2022, https:// www.cihi.ca/en/physicians-in-canada.
50 Canadian Institute for Health Information, "Physicians."
51 Marilou Gagnon and Amélie Perron, "Nursing Voices during COVID-19: An Analysis of Canadian Media Coverage," *Aporia: The Nursing Journal* 12, no. 1 (2020): 109–13, https://doi.org/10.18192/aporia.v12i1 .4842.
52 Andrea C. Tricco et al., "Advancing Gender Equity in Medicine," *CMAJ* 193, no. 7 (2021): e244–50, https://doi.org/10.1503/cmaj.200951.
53 Oveisi et al., "The Experiences of Nurses in British Columbia," 6.
54 Canadian Institute for Health Information, "COVID-19 Cases and Deaths in Health Care Workers in Canada."
55 Oveisi et al., "The Experiences of Nurses in British Columbia," 4.

Chapter 17: #InItTogether Is Only a Hashtag for Canadian Caregivers

1 Statistics Canada, "Caregivers in Canada, 2018," last updated 10 January 2020, https://www150.statcan.gc.ca/n1/daily-quotidien/200108 /dq200108a-eng.htm.
2 Angus Reid, "Caregiving in Canada: As Population Ages, One-in-Four Canadians Over 30 Are Looking After Loved Ones," 12 August 2019, https://angusreid.org/wp-content/uploads/2019/08/2019.08.12 _Caregiving.pdf.

3 Elder Abuse Prevention Ontario, "National Caregiver Day: Recognizing Caring Canadians," accessed 9 June 2023, https://eapon.ca/recognizing-caring-canadians/.
4 Canadian Centre for Caregiving Excellence, "Caregiver Resources," accessed 9 June 2023, https://canadiancaregiving.org/caregivers/caregiver-resources/.

Chapter 19: The Levee Has Broken

1 Ontario Nurses' Association, "Learn about ONA's Fight to Defeat Bill 124," accessed 11 June 2023, https://www.ona.org/about-bill-124/.
2 SIEU Healthcare, "Ford Government Must Stop Attacks on Healthcare Workers," 13 July 2020, https://seiuhealthcare.ca/ford-government-must-stop-attacks-on-healthcare-workers/.
3 Canadian Institute for Health Information, *Nursing in Canada, 2018: A Lens on Supply and Workforce* (Ottawa: CIHI, 2019), https://www.cihi.ca/sites/default/files/document/regulated-nurses-2018-report-en-web.pdf.
4 World Health Organization, "Year of the Nurse and the Midwife, 2020," https://www.who.int/campaigns/annual-theme/year-of-the-nurse-and-the-midwife-2020.

Chapter 20: "We're All in This Together"

1 *High School Musical*, 2006, IMDb, https://www.imdb.com/title/tt0475293/.
2 António Guterres, "We Are All in This Together: Human Rights and COVID-19 Response and Recovery," United Nations, 23 April 2020, https://www.un.org/en/un-coronavirus-communications-team/we-are-all-together-human-rights-and-covid-19-response-and.
3 Ryan Nolan, "'We Are All in This Together!' COVID-19 and the Lie of Solidarity," *Irish Journal of Sociology* 29, no. 1 (2020): 102–6, https://doi.org/10.1177/0791603520940967.
4 United States Environmental Protection Agency, "Learn about Environmental Justice," last updated 6 September 2022, https://www.epa.gov/environmentaljustice/learn-about-environmental-justice#:~:text=President%20Clinton%20signing%20the%20EJ,environmental%20laws%2C%20regulations%20and%20policies.
5 Dalia Hasan (@DaliaHasanMD), "In one emoji, here's what I think about 'pandemic amnesty' and 'you do you,'" Twitter, 1 November 2022, 8:01 p.m., https://twitter.com/DaliaHasanMD/status/1587595690431086593?s=20&t=2Fr44y9MDukZJuWr4bByvg.
6 Environmental Justice/Environmental Racism, "Principles of Environmental Justice," last updated 6 April 1996, https://www.ejnet.org/ej/principles.html.
7 Environmental Justice/Environmental Racism, "Principles."
8 Parliament of Canada, "Strengthening Environmental Protection for a Healthier Canada Act," accessed 13 June 2023, https://www.parl.ca/legisinfo/en/bill/44-1/s-5.

9 United Nations, "Climate and Environment," 28 July 2022, https://news .un.org/en/story/2022/07/1123482.

10 Parliament of Canada, "National Strategy Respecting Environmental Racism and Environmental Justice Act," accessed 13 June 2023, https:// www.parl.ca/legisinfo/en/bill/44-1/c-226.

11 Jane Elizabeth McArthur, "Dichotomies, Transcendence and Power: Investigating Women's Narratives of Breast Cancer Risks" (PhD diss., University of Windsor, 2021), https://scholar.uwindsor.ca/etd/8567/.

12 Janet M. Gray et al., "State of the Evidence 2017: An Update on the Connection between Breast Cancer and the Environment," *Environmental Health* 16, no. 94 (2017), https://doi.org/10.1186/s12940-017-0287-4.

13 David Kriebel, "The Precautionary Principle in Environmental Science," *Environmental Health Perspectives* 109, no. 9 (2001): 871–6, https://doi .org/10.1289/ehp.01109871.

14 Jane E. McArthur, "Blaming Women for Breast Cancer Ignores Environmental Risk Factors," *The Conversation*, 21 June 2020, https:// theconversation.com/blaming-women-for-breast-cancer-ignores -environmental-risk-factors-139719.

15 Jane E. McArthur, "As the Oceans Rise, So Do Your Risks of Breast Cancer," *The Conversation*, 15 January 2019, https://theconversation.com /as-the-oceans-rise-so-do-your-risks-of-breast-cancer-108420.

16 The BTL Editorial Committee, *Sick of the System: Why the COVID-19 Recovery Must Be Revolutionary* (Toronto: Between the Lines, 2020), https:// www.uwindsor.ca/sociology/sites/uwindsor.ca.sociology/files/novel _virus_old_story_sickofthesystem_mcarthurbrophykeith.pdf.

17 Jane McArthur, "Guest Column: Without All the Evidence on COVID-19, Use the Precautionary Principle," *Windsor Star*, 13 April 2020, https:// windsorstar.com/opinion/columnists/guest-column-without-all-the -evidence-on-covid-19-use-the-precautionary-principle.

18 Jane McArthur and Filipe Duarte, "Prioritizing Collective Responsibilities in the Response to COVID-19," *Canadian Dimension*, 17 April 2020, https://canadiandimension.com/articles/view/prioritizing-collective -responsibilities-in-the-response-to-covid-19.

19 Renyi Zang et al., "Identifying Airborne Transmission as the Dominant Route for the Spread of COVID-19," *PNAS* 117, no. 26 (2020): 14857–63, https://doi.org/10.1073/pnas.2009637117.

20 Columbia Law School, "Kimberlé Crenshaw on Intersectionality, More than Two Decades Later," 8 June 2017, https://www.law.columbia.edu /news/archive/kimberle-crenshaw-intersectionality-more-two-decades -later.

21 James T. Brophy et al., "Sacrificed: Ontario Healthcare Workers in the Time of COVID-19," *NEW SOLUTIONS: A Journal of Environmental and Occupational Health Policy* 30, no. 4 (2021): 267–81, https://doi .org/10.1177/1048291120974358.

22 Ontario Council of Hospital Unions and Canadian Union of Public Employees, "International Researchers Call for an End to the Sacrifice of Health Care Workers," 25 April 2021, https://ochu.on.ca/2021/04/25

/international-researchers-call-for-an-end-to-the-sacrifice-of-health-care
-workers/.

23 The SARS Commission, *Final Report*, December 2006, http://www
.archives.gov.on.ca/en/e_records/sars/index.html.

24 OCHU and CUPE, "International Researchers," 2.

25 Barry Hunt (@BarryHunt008), "1. Concentration of SARS2 virus in air
is higher in less well ventilated spaces," Twitter, 5 April 2023, 9:25 a.m.,
https://twitter.com/BarryHunt008/status/1643605756053258240?s=20.

26 Health Canada, *Health Impacts of Air Pollution in Canada: Estimates of
Morbidity and Premature Mortality Outcomes – 2021 Report* (Ottawa:
Health Canada, 2021), https://www.canada.ca/en/health-canada/services
/publications/healthy-living/2021-health-effects-indoor-air-pollution.html.

27 Cathryn Tonne et al., "Socioeconomic and Ethnic Inequalities in Exposure
to Air and Noise Pollution in London," *Environmental International* 115
(2018): 170–9, https://doi.org/10.1016/j.envint.2018.03.023.

28 Chen Chen et al., "Association between Long-Term Exposure to Ambi-
ent Air Pollution and COVID-19 Severity: A Prospective Cohort Study,"
CMAJ 194, no. 20 (24 May 2022): e693–700, https://doi.org/10.1503/cmaj
.220068.

29 Canadian Association of Physicians for the Environment, *Mobilizing Evidence: Activating Change on Traffic-Related Air Pollution (TRAP)
Health Impacts* (Toronto: CAPE, 2021), https://cape.ca/wp-content
/uploads/2022/05/CAPE-TRAP-2022-2.pdf.

30 Zander S. Venter, "COVID-19 Lockdowns Cause Global Air Pollution
Declines," *PNAS* 117, no. 32 (2020): 18984–90, https://doi.org/10.1073
/pnas.2006853117.

31 University of California, Davis, Environmental Health, "Race, COVID-19,
and Air Pollution," accessed 13 June 2023, https://environmentalhealth
.ucdavis.edu/sites/g/files/dgvnsk2556/files/media/documents
/Air%20pollution%2C%20race%20%26%20COVID-19.pdf.

32 John Parsons, "About," http://jonparsons.ca/.

33 Nancy Krieger and Anne-Emmanuelle Birn, "A Vision of Social Justice as
the Foundation of Public Health: Commemorating 150 Years of the Spirit
of 1848," *American Journal of Public Health* 88, no. 11 (1998): 1603–733,
https://ajph.aphapublications.org/doi/epdf/10.2105/AJPH.88.11.1603.

34 Ted Schettler, "Toward an Ecological View of Health: An Imperative for
the Twenty-First Century" (paper presented by The Center for Health
Design and Health Care without Harm at a conference sponsored
by the Robert Wood Johnson Foundation, September 2006), https://
www.healthdesign.org/chd/research/toward-ecological-view-health
-imperative-twenty-first-century.

35 Urie Bronfenbrenner, "Ecological Models of Human Development,"
Readings on the Development of Children, 2nd ed., ed. Mary Gauvain and
Michael Cole (New York: Freeman, 1993), 37–43, https://impactof
specialneeds.weebly.com/uploads/3/4/1/9/3419723/ecologial_models
_of_human_development.pdf.

36 Christine Sismondo, "Why a Top Notch Air Exchanger Is Way More Effective than Plexiglas When It Comes to Good Ventilation," *Toronto Star*, 11 October 2021, https://www.thestar.com/life/health_wellness/advice/2021/10/11/why-a-top-notch-air-exchanger-is-way-more-effective-than-plexiglas-when-it-comes-to-good-ventilation.html.
37 "UN General Assembly Declares Access to Clean and Healthy Environment a Universal Human Right," UN News, 28 July 2022, https://news.un.org/en/story/2022/07/1123482.
38 Raina Delisle, "'I Can Feel Your Breath': When COVID-19 and Environmental Racism Collide," *The Narwhal*, 19 March 2021, https://thenarwhal.ca/covid-19-environmental-racism-canada/.

Chapter 22: The Doctor as Advocate

1 *Merriam-Webster Dictionary Online*, s.v. "advocacy," accessed 14 June 2023, https://www.merriam-webster.com/dictionary/advocacy.
2 Ableism: Social habits, practices, regulations, laws, and institutions that operate under the assumption that disabled people are inherently less capable overall, less valuable in society, and/or should have less personal autonomy than is ordinarily granted to people of the same age. See Andrew Pulrang, "Words Matter, and It's Time to Explore the Meaning of 'Ableism,'" *Forbes*, 25 October 2020 https://www.forbes.com/sites/andrewpulrang/2020/10/25/words-matter-and-its-time-to-explore-the-meaning-of-ableism/?sh=cd202897162d.
3 The SARS Commission, *Final Report*, December 2006, http://www.archives.gov.on.ca/en/e_records/sars/index.html.
4 World Health Organization, "Coronavirus Disease (COVID-19): How Is It Transmitted?," 23 December 2021, https://www.who.int/emergencies/diseases/novel-coronavirus-2019/question-and-answers-hub/q-a-detail/coronavirus-disease-covid-19-how-is-it-transmitted?gclid=CjwKCAjwq-WgBhBMEiwAzKSH6EnJS4TvAFq9cWi9x2DwYDZ8TPCK8pKmawZDBisIK3hYg1NTDCkQkBoC5hwQAvD_BwE.
5 Centers for Disease Control and Prevention, "Scientific Brief: SARS-CoV-2 Transmission," last updated 7 May 2021, https://www.cdc.gov/coronavirus/2019-ncov/science/science-briefs/sars-cov-2-transmission.html.
6 Public Health Agency of Canada, "COVID-19: Main Modes of Transmission," last updated 29 June 2021, https://www.canada.ca/en/public-health/services/diseases/2019-novel-coronavirus-infection/health-professionals/main-modes-transmission.html.
7 United Stated Environmental Protection Agency, "Indoor Air and Coronavirus (COVID-19)," last updated 7 June 2023, https://www.epa.gov/coronavirus/indoor-air-and-coronavirus-covid-19.
8 ASHRAE, "ASHRAE Epidemic Task Force Releases Updated Airborne Transmission Guidance," 5 April 2021, https://www.ashrae.org

/about/news/2021/ashrae-epidemic-task-force-releases-updated
-airborne-transmission-guidance.

9 The White House, "Let's Clear the Air on COVID," 23 March 2022,
https://www.whitehouse.gov/ostp/news-updates/2022/03/23
/lets-clear-the-air-on-covid/.

Chapter 23: Disability Rights and Advocacy

1 I received a reply from the Office of the Chief Medical Officer of Health
(CMOH) on 27 March 2023, which included twenty-nine PDF documents.
These included internal communications between the CMOH and other
senior government advisers and representatives. I prepared a thorough
analysis of the release and have shared it with opposition members of the
Ontario Legislative Assembly and others. The brief, "Stepping Away from
an Evidence-Based Public Health Policy and the Precautionary Principle
during the Time of Omicron: Did the Ontario Government Fail to Consider the Potential Harms to Highly COVID-19 Vulnerable Ontarians?"
is now available online (https://drive.google.com/file/d/1BkIVN8u1u
9G86q5LtNBvWVAgMM8S_Hj9/view?pli=1). It was my finding that
in 2022 the Ford government ignored advice from senior government
advisers from Public Health Ontario, the Ministry of Health, Medical
Officers of Health, and the Ontario COVID-19 Advisory Science Table for
more stringent public health measures, including the use of N95/KN95
masks in the community. The CMOH, the minister of health, and the
Office of the Premier provided little evidence whatsoever that the vulnerable were considered as they withdrew public health measures during
the deadliest year of the pandemic. My findings are summarized in "If
Public Health Is Not There to Protect the Vulnerable, Then Why Bother?"
Healthy Debate, 19 July 2023, https://healthydebate.ca/2023/07/topic
/public-health-not-protect-vulnerable/.

Chapter 24: "Truth"

1 Andrew Buncombe, "These Experts Say Joe Rogan Is 'Extraordinarily
Dangerous' to Society – Here's Why," *The Independent*, 27 January 2022,
https://www.independent.co.uk/news/world/americas/joe-rogan
-podcast-spotify-covid-malone-b2002301.html.

2 Ed Yong, "Why the Coronavirus Is So Confusing," *The Atlantic*, 29
April 2020, https://www.theatlantic.com/health/archive/2020/04
/pandemic-confusing-uncertainty/610819/.

Chapter 25: I Work in a Hospital

1 Bethany Lindsay, "False Claims of Stillbirths among Vaccinated Mothers at B.C. Hospital Slammed as Harmful Disinformation," *CBC News*, 24

November 2021, https://www.cbc.ca/news/canada/british-columbia
/covid19-vaccine-false-claims-stillbirth-1.6261062.
2 All names are pseudonyms.
3 Ashleigh Stewart, "Fact Check: COVID-19 Vaccines Are Not Causing a
   Rise in Stillbirths in Canada," *Global News*, 25 November 2021, https://
   globalnews.ca/news/8401613/fact-check-covid-19-vaccines-stillbirths
   -pregnancy/.

Chapter 26: How to Be Wrong

1 Johns Hopkins University Coronavirus Resource Centre, "Global Map,"
   accessed 13 September 2022, https://coronavirus.jhu.edu/map.html (the
   site stopped collecting data as of 10 March 2023).
2 Anonymous, "The Pandemic's True Death Toll: Our Daily Estimate of
   Excess Deaths around the World," *The Economist*, 21 September 2022,
   https://www.economist.com/graphic-detail/coronavirus-excess-deaths
   -estimates.
3 Amat Adarov, "Global Income Inequality and the COVID-19 Pandemic in Three Charts," *World Bank Blogs*, 7 February 2022, https://
   blogs.worldbank.org/developmenttalk/global-income-inequality-and
   -covid-19-pandemic-three-charts.
4 Susan D. Hillis et al., "Global Minimum Estimates of Children Affected
   by COVID-19–Associated Orphanhood and Deaths of Caregivers: A
   Modelling Study," *The Lancet* 398, no. 10298 (2021): 391–402, https://doi
   .org/10.1016/S0140-6736(21)01253-8.
5 Rochelle Knight et al., "Association of COVID-19 with Major Arterial and
   Venous Thrombotic Diseases: A Population-Wide Cohort Study of 48 Million Adults in England and Wales," *Circulation* 146, no. 12 (2022): 892–906,
   https://doi.org/10.1161/CIRCULATIONAHA.122.060785.
6 Andrea G. Edlow et al., "Neurodevelopmental Outcomes at 1 Year in Infants of Mothers Who Tested Positive for SARS-CoV-2 during Pregnancy,"
   JAMA Network Open 5, no. 6 (2022): e2215787, https://doi.org/10.1001
   /jamanetworkopen.2022.15787.
7 Eric J. Topol and Akiko Iwasaki, "Operation Nasal Vaccine – Light-
   ning Speed to Counter COVID-19," *Science Immunology* 7, no. 74 (2022):
   eadd9947, https://doi.org/10.1126/sciimmunol.add9947.
8 Thomas C. Williams et al., "Sensitivity of RT-PCR Testing of Upper Respiratory Tract Samples for SARS-CoV-2 in Hospitalised Patients: A Retrospective Cohort Study," *Welcome Open Research* 5, no. 254 (2020), https://
   doi.org/10.12688/wellcomeopenres.16342.2; Michael J. Mina et al.,
   "Clarifying the Evidence on SARS-CoV-2 Antigen Rapid Tests in Public
   Health Responses to COVID-19," *The Lancet* 397, no. 10283 (2021): 1425–7,
   https://doi.org/10.1016/S0140-6736(21)00425-6.
9 Lidia Morawska et al., "How Can Airborne Transmission of COVID-19
   Indoors Be Minimised?," *Environment International* 142 (2020): 105832,
   https://doi.org/10.1016/j.envint.2020.105832; Lidia Morawska and

Donald K. Milton, "It Is Time to Address Airborne Transmission of Coronavirus Disease 2019 (COVID-19)," *Clinical Infectious Diseases* 71, no. 9 (2020): 2311–3, https://doi.org/10.1093/cid/ciaa939; Kimberly A. Prather et al., "Airborne Transmission of SARS-CoV-2," *Science* 370, no. 6514 (2020): 303–4, https://www.science.org/doi/epdf/10.1126/science.abf0521.

10   Lara B. Aknin et al., "Policy Stringency and Mental Health during the COVID-19 Pandemic: A Longitudinal Analysis of Data from 15 Countries," *The Lancet Public Health* 7, no. 5 (2022): e417–26, https://doi.org/10.1016/S2468-2667(22)00060-3.

11   Valeria Trivellone, Eric P. Hoberg, Walter A. Boeger, and Daniel R. Brooks, "Food Security and Emerging Infectious Disease: Risk Assessment and Risk Management," *Royal Society Open Science* 9, no. 2 (2022): 211687, https://doi.org/10.1098/rsos.211687.

12   Max Kozlov, "Risky 'Gain-of-Function' Studies Need Stricter Guidance, Say US Researchers," *Nature* 605, no. 7909 (2022): 203–4, https://doi.org/10.1038/d41586-022-01209-w.

13   Jose L. Jimenez et al., "What Were the Historical Reasons for the Resistance to Recognizing Airborne Transmission during the COVID-19 Pandemic?," *Indoor Air* 32, no. 8 (2022): e13070, https://doi.org/10.1111/ina.13070; Katherine Randal et al., "How Did We Get Here: What Are Droplets and Aerosols and How Far Do They Go? A Historical Perspective on the Transmission of Respiratory Infectious Diseases," *Interface Focus* 11, no. 6 (2021): 20210049, https://doi.org/10.1098/rsfs.2021.0049.

14   J.N. Hays, "Cholera and Sanitation," in *The Burdens of Disease: Epidemics and Human Response in Western History*, 2nd ed. (New Brunswick, NJ: Rutgers University Press, 2009), 135–54.

15   Hays, "Cholera and Sanitation."

16   Hays, "Cholera and Sanitation."

17   Frank M. Snowden, "The Sanitary Movement," in *Epidemics and Society: From the Black Death to the Present* (New Haven, CT: Yale University Press, 2019), 184–203.

18   Hays, "Cholera and Sanitation"; Peter Vinten-Johansen et al., "Snow's Cholera Theory," in *Cholera, Chloroform, and the Science of Medicine: A Life of John Snow* (New York: Oxford University Press, 2003), 199–230; Peter Vinten-Johansen et al., "Professional Success," in *Cholera, Chloroform, and the Science of Medicine: A Life of John Snow* (New York: Oxford University Press, 2003), 231–53.

19   Ashleigh R. Tuite, Christina H. Chan, and David N. Fisman, "Cholera, Canals, and Contagion: Rediscovering Dr. Beck's Report," *Journal of Public Health Policy* 32, no. 3 (2011): 320–33, https://doi.org/10.1057/jphp.2011.20.

20   Tuite, Chan, and Fisman, "Cholera, Canals, and Contagion"; Ruth Richardson, "The Act Is Uninjurious if Unknown," *Death, Dissection and the Destitute* (Harmondsworth, UK: Penguin Books, 1988), 219–38.

21 Snowden, "The Sanitary Movement"; Peter Vinten-Johansen et al., "Professional Success."
22 Dana Tulodziecki, "A Case Study in Explanatory Power: John Snow's Conclusions about the Pathology and Transmission of Cholera," *Studies in History and Philosophy of Science Part C: Studies in History and Philosophy of Biological and Biomedical Sciences* 42, no. 3 (2011): 306–16, https://doi.org/10.1016/j.shpsc.2011.02.001.
23 Tuite, Chan, and Fisman, "Cholera, Canals, and Contagion."
24 Peter Vinten-Johansen et al., "Ether," in *Cholera, Chloroform, and the Science of Medicine: A Life of John Snow* (New York: Oxford University Press, 2003), 110–39.
25 Peter Vinten-Johansen et al., "Snow and the Mapping of Cholera Epidemics," in *Cholera, Chloroform, and the Science of Medicine: A Life of John Snow* (New York: Oxford University Press, 2003), 318–39.
26 Tulodziecki, "A Case Study in Explanatory Power."
27 Vinten-Johansen et al., "Snow's Cholera Theory"; Tulodziecki, "A Case Study in Explanatory Power."
28 Vinten-Johansen et al., "Snow's Cholera Theory."
29 Peter Vinten-Johansen et al., "Snow and the Sanitarians," in *Cholera, Chloroform, and the Science of Medicine: A Life of John Snow* (New York: Oxford University Press, 2003), 340–58.
30 Peter Vinten-Johansen et al., "Snow's Multiple Legacies," in *Cholera, Chloroform, and the Science of Medicine: A Life of John Snow* (New York: Oxford University Press, 2003), 388–403.
31 Jimenez et al., "What Were the Historical Reasons"; Randal et al., "How Did We Get Here."
32 William F. Wells and Mildred W. Wells, "Air-Borne Infection," *JAMA* 107, no. 21 (1936): 1698–703, https://doi.org/10.1001/jama.1936.02770470016004; William F. Wells, "On Air-Borne Infection: Study II. Droplets and Droplet Nuclei," *American Journal of Epidemiology* 20, no. 3 (1934): 611–18, https://doi.org/10.1093/oxfordjournals.aje.a118097.
33 J.W. Tang et al., "Dismantling Myths on the Airborne Transmission of Severe Acute Respiratory Syndrome Coronavirus-2 (SARS-CoV-2)," *Journal of Hospital Infection* 110 (2021): 89–96, https://doi.org/10.1016/j.jhin.2020.12.022.
34 Justice Archer et al., "Comparing Aerosol Number and Mass Exhalation Rates from Children and Adults during Breathing, Speaking and Singing," *Interface Focus* 12, no. 2 (2022): 20210078, https://doi.org/10.1098/rsfs.2021.0078; Christopher M. Orton et al., "A Comparison of Respiratory Particle Emission Rates at Rest and while Speaking or Exercising," *Communications Medicine* 2 (2022): article 44, https://doi.org/10.1038/s43856-022-00103-w.
35 Richard L. Riley et al., "Infectiousness of Air from a Tuberculosis Ward. Ultraviolet Irradiation of Infected Air: Comparative Infectiousness of Different Patients," *American Review of Respiratory Disease* 85, no. 4 (1962): 511–25, https://pubmed.ncbi.nlm.nih.gov/14492300/.

36 Jimenez et al., "What Were the Historical Reasons"; Randal et al., "How Did We Get Here."
37 Jimenez et al., "What Were the Historical Reasons."
38 Tang et al., "Dismantling Myths on the Airborne Transmission."
39 Public Health Agency of Canada, *Routine Practices and Additional Precautions for Preventing the Transmission of Infection in Healthcare Settings* (Ottawa: Minister of Public Works and Government Services, 2016), https://www.canada.ca/content/dam/phac-aspc/documents/services/publications/diseases-conditions/routine-practices-precautions-healthcare-associated-infections/routine-practices-precautions-healthcare-associated-infections-2016-FINAL-eng.pdf; US Centers for Disease Control and Prevention, "Background C. Air: Guidelines for Environmental Infection Control in Health-Care Facilities (2003)," Infection Control, last updated 22 July 2019, https://www.cdc.gov/infectioncontrol/guidelines/environmental/background/air.html#c2.
40 Edward A. Nardell, "Air Disinfection for Airborne Infection Control with a Focus on COVID-19: Why Germicidal UV Is Essential," special issue dedicated to the topics of germicidal photobiology and infection control, *Photochemistry and Photobiology* 97, no. 3 (2021): 493–7, https://doi.org/10.1111/php.13421.
41 X. Wang, Z. Pan, and Z. Cheng, "Association between 2019-nCoV Transmission and N95 Respirator Use," *Journal of Hospital Infection* 105, no. 1 (2020): 104–5, https://doi.org/10.1016/j.jhin.2020.02.021.
42 Mieli Li et al., "Transmission Characteristics of the COVID-19 Outbreak in China: A Study Driven by Data," *medRxiv* (preprint, submitted in 2020), https://doi.org/10.1101/2020.02.26.20028431.
43 Parham Azimi et al., "Mechanistic Transmission Modeling of COVID-19 on the *Diamond Princess* Cruise Ship Demonstrates the Importance of Aerosol Transmission," *PNAS* 118, no. 8 (2021): e2015482118, https://doi.org/10.1073/pnas.2015482118; G. Correia, L. Rodrigues, M. Gameiro da Silva, and T. Goncalves, "Airborne Route and Bad Use of Ventilation Systems as Non-Negligible Factors in SARS-CoV-2 Transmission," *Medical Hypotheses* 141 (2020): 109781, https://doi.org/10.1016/j.mehy.2020.109781; Shelly L. Miller et al., "Transmission of SARS-CoV-2 by Inhalation of Respiratory Aerosol in the Skagit Valley Chorale Superspreading Event," *Indoor Air* 31, no. 2 (2021): 314–23, https://doi.org/10.1111/ina.12751; Hiroshi Nishiura et al., "Closed Environments Facilitate Secondary Transmission of Coronavirus Disease 2019 (COVID-19)," *medRxiv* (preprint, submitted in 2020), https://doi.org/10.1101/2020.02.28.20029272; Trisha Greenhalgh et al., "Ten Scientific Reasons in Support of Airborne Transmission of SARS-CoV-2," *The Lancet* 397, no. 10285 (2021): P1603–5, https://doi.org/10.1016/S0140-6736(21)00869-2.
44 Morawska and Milton, "It Is Time to Address Airborne Transmission."
45 Zain Chagla, Susy Hota, Sarah Khan, and Dominik Mertz, "Re: It Is Time to Address Airborne Transmission of COVID-19," *Clinical Infectious Diseases* 73, no. 11 (2021): e3981–2, https://doi.org/10.1093/cid/ciaa1118.

46 Qun Li et al., "Early Transmission Dynamics in Wuhan, China, of Novel Coronavirus-Infected Pneumonia," *New England Journal of Medicine* 382, no. 13 (2020): 1199–207, https://www.nejm.org/doi/10.1056/nejmoa 2001316.

47 Pandemic Influenza Outbreak Research Modelling Team (Pan-InfORM), "Modelling an Influenza Pandemic: A Guide for the Perplexed," *CMAJ* 181, no. 3–4 (2009): 171–3, https://doi.org/10.1503/cmaj.090885.

48 Jenna Gettings et al., "Mask Use and Ventilation Improvements to Reduce COVID-19 Incidence in Elementary Schools – Georgia, November 16–December 11, 2020," *Morbidity and Mortality Weekly Report (MMWR)* 70, no. 21 (2021): 779–84, https://doi.org/10.15585/mmwr.mm7021e1.

49 Kristin L. Andrejko et al., "Effectiveness of Face Mask or Respirator Use in Indoor Public Settings for Prevention of SARS-CoV-2 Infection – California, February–December 2021," *Morbidity and Mortality Weekly Report (MMWR)* 71, no. 6 (2022): 212–16, https://doi.org/10.15585/mmwr.mm7106e1.

50 Jeffrey D. Sachs et al., "The *Lancet* Commission on Lessons for the Future from the COVID-19 Pandemic," *The Lancet Commissions* 400, no. 10359 (2022): P1224–80, https://doi.org/10.1016/S0140-6736(22)01585-9.

51 Erica Weir, Richard Schabas, Kumanan Wilson, and Chris Mackie, "A Canadian Framework for Applying the Precautionary Principle to Public Health Issues," *Canadian Journal of Public Health* 101, no. 5 (2010): 396–8, https://doi.org/10.1007/BF03404860; Kumanan Wilson, "The Krever Commission – 10 Years Later," *CMAJ* 177, no. 11 (2007): 1387–9, https://doi.org/10.1503/cmaj.071333.

52 Lok Bahadur Shrestha et al., "Evolution of the SARS-CoV-2 Omicron Variants BA.1 to BA.5: Implications for Immune Escape and Transmission," *Reviews in Medical Virology* 32, no. 5 (2022): e2381, https://doi .org/10.1002/rmv.2381; Pooja Khairnar et al., "Recent Highlights on Omicron as a New SARS-COVID-19 Variant: Evolution, Genetic Mutation, and Future Perspectives," *Journal of Drug Targeting* 30, no. 6 (2022): 603–13, https://doi.org/10.1080/1061186x.2022.2056187.

53 Miguel Padilla-Blanco et al., "The Finding of the Severe Acute Respiratory Syndrome Coronavirus (SARS-CoV-2) in a Wild Eurasian River Otter (*Lutra lutra*) Highlights the Need for Viral Surveillance in Wild Mustelids," *Frontiers in Veterinary Science* 9 (2022): 826991, https://doi .org/10.3389/fvets.2022.82699; M. Pomorska-Mol, J. Wlodarek, M. Gogulski, and M. Rybska, "Review: SARS-CoV-2 Infection in Farmed Minks – An Overview of Current Knowledge on Occurrence, Disease and Epidemiology," *Animal* 15, no. 7 (2021): 100272, https://doi.org/10.1016/j .animal.2021.100272; Slavoljub Stanojevicet et al., "Frequency of SARS-CoV-2 Infection in Dogs and Cats: Results of a Retrospective Serological Survey in Sumadija District, Serbia," *Preventive Veterinary Medicine* 208 (2022): 105755, https://doi.org/10.1016/j.prevetmed.2022.105755.

54 Roger A. Pielke Jr., "Science and Decision-Making," in *The Honest Broker: Making Sense of Science in Policy and Politics* (Cambridge: Cambridge University Press, 2007), 23–38; Roger A. Pielke Jr., "Making Sense of Science

in Policy and Politics," in *The Honest Broker: Making Sense of Science in Policy and Politics* (Cambridge: Cambridge University Press, 2007), 135–52.

55 Pielke Jr., "Science and Decision-Making"; and Pielke Jr., "Making Sense of Science in Policy and Politics."

56 Pielke Jr., "Science and Decision-Making"; and Pielke Jr., "Making Sense of Science in Policy and Politics."

57 Paul Dolan, "Utilitarianism and the Measurement and Aggregation of Quality – Adjusted Life Years," *Health Care Analysis* 9, no. 1 (2001): 65–76, https://doi.org/10.1023/A:1011387524579.

58 Aknin et al., "Policy Stringency and Mental Health."

59 Liz Frazier, "The Coronavirus Crash of 2020, and the Investing Lesson It Taught Us," *Forbes*, 11 February 2021, https://www.forbes.com/sites/lizfrazierpeck/2021/02/11/the-coronavirus-crash-of-2020-and-the-investing-lesson-it-taught-us/?sh=7e22abba46cf.

60 Press Progress, "Company Hired to Manage Ontario's COVID-19 School Reopening Highlighted Business Opportunities for Private Education Providers," 21 July 2021, https://pressprogress.ca/company-hired-to-manage-ontarios-covid-19-school-reopening-highlighted-business-opportunities-for-private-education-providers/; Thomas Gerbet, "Dans l'ombre, la firme McKinsey était au cœur de la gestion de la pandémie au Québec," *Radio Canada*, 30 September 2022, https://ici.radio-canada.ca/nouvelle/1920666/mckinsey-quebec-covid-legault-gestion-pandemie.

61 Tara Kirk Sell et al., *National Priorities to Combat Misinformation and Disinformation for COVID-19 and Future Public Health Threats: A Call for a National Strategy* (Baltimore: Johns Hopkins Center for Health Security, 2021), https://centerforhealthsecurity.org/sites/default/files/2023-02/210322-misinformation.pdf.

62 Natasha Ruth Saunders et al., "Changes in Hospital-Based Care Seeking for Acute Mental Health Concerns among Children and Adolescents during the COVID-19 Pandemic in Ontario, Canada, through September 2021," *JAMA Network Open* 5, no. 7 (2022): e2220553, https://doi.org/10.1001/jamanetworkopen.2022.20553; Joel G. Ray et al., "Comparison of Self-Harm or Overdose among Adolescents and Young Adults before vs during the COVID-19 Pandemic in Ontario," *JAMA Network Open* 5, no. 1 (2022): e2143144, https://doi.org/10.1001/jamanetworkopen.2021.43144.

63 Trisha Greenhalgh et al., "Adapt or Die: How the Pandemic Made the Shift from EBM to EBM+ More Urgent," *BMJ Evidence-Based Medicine* 17, no. 5 (2022), https://doi.org/10.1136/bmjebm-2022-111952.

64 Ingela Alger and Jörgen W. Weibull, "Strategic Behavior of Moralists and Altruists," special issue on ethics, morality, and game theory, *Games* 8, no. 3 (2017): 38, https://doi.org/10.3390/g8030038.

65 Shikha Gupta and Nicole Aitken, "COVID-19 Mortality among Racialized Populations in Canada and Its Association with Income," Statistics Canada, 30 August 2022, https://www150.statcan.gc.ca/n1/pub/45-28-0001/2022001/article/00010-eng.htm.

66 Morawska et al., "How Can Airborne Transmission of COVID-19 Indoors Be Minimised?"; Nardell, "Air Disinfection for Airborne Infection Control."

Printed in the USA
CPSIA information can be obtained
at www.ICGtesting.com
CBHW020807291024
16365CB00035B/74